WHO Technical Report Series
925

EVALUATION OF CERTAIN VETERINARY DRUG RESIDUES IN FOOD

Sixty-second report of the
Joint FAO/WHO Expert Committee on
Food Additives

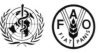

D0770581

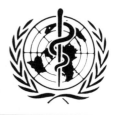

World Health Organization
Geneva 2004

WHO Library Cataloguing-in-Publication Data

Joint FAO/WHO Expert Committee on Food Additives (2004 : Rome, Italy)
    Evaluation of certain food additives and contaminants : sixty-second report of the
    Joint FAO/WHO Expert Committee on Food Additives.

    (WHO technical report series; 925)

    1.Food contamination 2.Drug residues — analysis 3.Drug residues — toxicity
    4.Veterinary drugs — toxicity 5.Risk assessment 6.Maximum allowable concentration —
    standards 7.No-observed-adverse-effect level

    I.Title II.Series

    ISBN 92 4 120925 9   (NLM Classification: WA 712)

    ISSN 0512-3054

Typeset in Hong Kong
Printed in Switzerland

Contents

1. Introduction   1

2. General considerations   2
    2.1 Conclusions on specific toxicological end-points   2
    2.2 Lipid-soluble residues of veterinary drugs with MRLs in milk   2
    2.3 Statistical methods for the estimation of MRLs   3
    2.4 Terminology for analytical methods (from the Codex Committee
         on Methods of Analysis and Sampling)   4
    2.5 Response to the Codex Committee on Residues of Veterinary
         Drugs in Foods on its Draft Risk Assessment Policy   5

3. Comments on residues of specific veterinary drugs   6
    3.1 Cefuroxime   7
    3.2 Cyhalothrin   10
    3.3 Cypermethrin and α-cypermethrin   12
    3.4 Doramectin   15
    3.5 Flumequine   18
    3.6 Lincomycin   21
    3.7 Melengestrol acetate   22
    3.8 Phoxim   25
    3.9 Pirlimycin   26
    3.10 Ractopamine   37

4. Comments on chloramphenicol found at low levels in animal products   49

5. Future work   56

6. Recommendations   57

Acknowledgement   58

References   58

Annex 1
Reports and other documents resulting from previous meetings of the
Joint FAO/WHO Expert Committee on Food Additives   59

Annex 2
Recommendations on compounds on the agenda   68

Sixty-second meeting of the Joint FAO/WHO Expert Committee o Food Additives

Rome, 4–12 February 2004

Members

Dr D. Arnold, Consultant, Berlin, Germany *(Chairman)*

Professor A.R. Boobis, Experimental Medicine and Toxicology, Division of Medicine, Faculty of Medicine, Imperial College, London, England

Dr R. Ellis, Senior Regulatory Scientist, Division of Human Food Safety, Office of New Animal Drug Evaluation, Center for Veterinary Medicine, Food and Drug Administration, Rockville, MD, USA

Dr A. Fernández Suárez, Instituto Nacional de Tecnología Agropecuaria Centro de Agroalimentos, Buenos Aires, Argentina

Dr K. Greenlees, Toxicologist, Division of Human Food Safety, Office of New Animal Drug Evaluation, Center for Veterinary Medicine, Food and Drug Administration, Rockville, MD, USA

Dr L.D.B. Kinabo, Dept. of Veterinary Physiology, Biochemistry, Pharmacology and Toxicology, Faculty of Veterinary Medicine, Sokoine University of Agriculture, Morogoro, Chuo Kikuu, United Republic of Tanzania

Dr J. MacNeil, Centre for Veterinary Drug Residues, Canadian Food Inspection Agency, Saskatoon Laboratory, Saskatoon, Saskatchewan, Canada

Professor J.G. McLean, Professor Emeritus, Camberwell, Victoria, Australia *(Vice-Chairman)*

Professor E.S. Mitema, Department of Public Health, Pharmacology and Toxicology, Faculty of Veterinary Medicine, College of Agriculture and Veterinary Sciences, University of Nairobi, Kabete, Kenya

Dr G. Moulin, Agence Française de Sécurité Sanitaire des Aliments, Agence Nationale du Médicament vétérinaire, Fougères, France

Professor J. Palermo-Neto, Department of Pathology, Faculty of Veterinary Medicine, University of São Paulo, São Paulo, Brazil

Dr J.L. Rojas Martínez, Ministerio de Agricultura y Ganadería, Laboratorio Nacional de Servicios Veterinarios, Barreal de Heredia, Heredia, Costa Rica

Dr S. Soback, Kimron Veterinary Institute, Ministry of Agriculture, Department of Residue Control and Food Hygiene, Beit Dagan, Israel

Secretariat

Dr C.E. Cerniglia, Director, Division of Microbiology, National Center for Toxicological Research, Food and Drug Administration, Jefferson, AR, USA (*WHO Temporary Adviser*)

Dr P. Chamberlain, Principal Scientist, Department of Toxicology, Covance Laboratories, Vienna, VA, USA (*WHO Temporary Adviser*)

Dr L.G. Friedlander, Leader, Residue Chemistry Team, Division of Human Food Safety, Office of New Animal Drug Evaluation, Center for Veterinary Medicine, Food and Drug Administration, Rockville, MD, USA (*FAO Consultant*)

Dr Z. Hailemariam, Head, Food Safety and Beverage Quality Control, Hygiene and Environmental Health Department Quality Control, Federal Ministry of Health, Addis Ababa, Ethiopia (*FAO Consultant*)

Dr J. Lewicki, Division of Pharmacology and Toxicology, Department of Preclinical Sciences, Faculty of Veterinary Medicine, Warsaw Agricultural University, Warsaw, Poland (*FAO Consultant*)

Dr M. Luetzow, Food Quality and Standards Service, Food and Nutrition Division, Food and Agriculture Organization of the United Nations, Rome, Italy (*FAO Joint Secretary*)

Dr Y. Ohno, Division of Pharmacology, Biological Safety Research Centre, National Institute of Health Sciences, Tokyo, Japan (*WHO Temporary Adviser*)

Dr S. Phongvivat, Food and Nutrition Division, Food and Agriculture Organization of the United Nations, Rome, Italy, (*FAO Visiting Scientist*)

Mrs I.M.E.J. Pronk, Center for Substances and Integrated Risk Assessment, National Institute for Public Health and the Environment, Bilthoven, The Netherlands (*WHO Temporary Adviser*)

Dr F. Ramos, Laboratório de Bromatologia, Nutrição e Hidrologia, Faculdade de Farmácia, Universidade de Coimbra, Coimbra, Portugal (*FAO Consultant*)

Dr P.T. Reeves, Australian Pesticides and Veterinary Medicines Authority, Kingston, ACT, Australia (*FAO Consultant*)

Mr D. Renshaw, Food Standards Agency, London, England (*WHO Temporary Adviser*)

Professor L. Ritter, Executive Director, Canadian Network of Toxicology Centres, Department of Environmental Biology, University of Guelph, Ontario, Canada (*WHO Temporary Adviser*)

Dr G. Roberts, Team Leader, Science Strategy (Veterinary), Therapeutic Goods Administration, Commonwealth Department of Health and Ageing, Woden, Australia (*WHO Temporary Adviser*)

Professor G.E. Swan, Department of Paraclinical Sciences, Faculty of Veterinary Science, University of Pretoria, Pretoria, South Africa (*FAO Consultant*)

Dr A. Tritscher, International Programme on Chemical Safety, World Health Organization, Geneva, Switzerland (*WHO Joint Secretary*)

Professor F.R. Ungemach, Institute of Pharmacology, Pharmacy and Toxicology, Faculty of Veterinary Medicine, University of Leipzig, Leipzig, Germany (*WHO Temporary Adviser*)

Dr J. Wongtavatchai, Department of Medicine, Faculty of Veterinary Science, Chulalongkorn University, Bangkok, Thailand (*WHO Temporary Adviser*)

Monographs containing summaries of relevant data and toxicological evaluations are available from WHO under the title:

Toxicological evaluation of certain veterinary drug residues in food. WHO Food Additive Series, No. 53, in preparation

Residues monographs are issued separately by FAO under the title:

Residues of some veterinary drugs in animals and foods, FAO Food and Nutrition Paper, No. 41/16, 2004.

INTERNATIONAL PROGRAMME ON CHEMICAL SAFETY

The preparatory work for toxicological evaluations of food additives and contaminants by the Joint FAO/WHO Expert Committee on Food Additives (JECFA) is actively supported by certain of the Member States that contribute to the work of the International Programme On Chemical Safety (IPCS). The IPCS is a joint venture of the United Nations Environment Programme, the International Labour Organisation and the World Health Organization. One of the main objectives of the IPCS is to carry out and disseminate evaluations of the effects of chemicals on human health and the quality of the environment.

---

1. Introduction

A meeting of the Joint FAO/WHO Expert Committee on Food Additives (JECFA) was held at the Food and Agriculture Organization of the United Nations (FAO) Headquarters, Rome, from 4 to 12 February 2004. The meeting was opened by Mr H. de Haen, Assistant Director-General, FAO, on behalf of the Directors-General of FAO and the World Health Organization (WHO). Mr de Haen referred to recent trade problems caused by food commodities containing substances that have no acceptable daily intake (ADI) or maximum residue limit (MRL). Mr de Haen noted that the Committee's deliberations on chloramphenicol would constitute an important input to a FAO/WHO technical workshop, established at the request of the Codex Alimentarius Commission, that would investigate the scientific and regulatory issues related to the risk analysis of substances without ADI or MRL.

Fifteen meetings of the Committee had been held to consider veterinary drug residues in food (Annex 1, references *80*, *85*, *91*, *97*, *104*, *110*, *113*, *119*, *125*, *128*, *134*, *140*, *146*, *157* and *163*) in response to the recommendations of a Joint FAO/WHO Expert Consultation held in 1984 (*1*). The present meeting[1] was convened in response to a recommendation made at the sixtieth meeting of the Committee (Annex 1, reference *163*) that meetings on this subject should be held regularly. The Committee's purpose was to provide guidance to FAO and WHO Member States and to the Codex Alimentarius Commission on public health issues pertaining to residues of veterinary drugs in foods of animal origin. The specific tasks before the Committee were:

— To elaborate further principles for evaluating the safety of residues of veterinary drugs in food, for establishing ADIs, and for recommending MRLs for such residues when the drugs under consideration are administered to food-producing animals in accordance with good practice in the use of veterinary drugs (see section 2); and
— To evaluate the safety of residues of certain veterinary drugs (see section 3 and Annex 2).
— To evaluate the safety of low levels of chloramphenicol in foods (section 4).

---

[1] As a result of the recommendations of the first Joint FAO/WHO Conference on Food Additives held in 1955 (FAO Nutrition Meeting Report Series, No. 11, 1956; WHO Technical Report Series, No. 107, 1956), there have been sixty-one previous meetings of the Joint FAO/WHO Expert Committee on Food Additives (Annex 1).

2. General considerations

2.1 Conclusions on specific toxicological end-points

In an effort to improve consistency and transparency, the Committee recommended that a series of standard statements be developed that allow clear and consistent conclusions to be expressed for specific toxicological end-points, in particular, genotoxic and carcinogenic potential, as well as reproductive toxicity. The Committee noted that the Joint FAO/WHO Meeting on Pesticide Residues (JMPR) has developed a set of statements that link these end-points to defined circumstances and that these statements should be used as a starting point and adapted and/or expanded as appropriate.

The Committee recommended that a small working group, including members of JECFA and JMPR Expert Committees, should elaborate a set of phrases to be used to describe the Committee's conclusions on genotoxic and carcinogenic potentials, for discussion at the next meetings, and taking into consideration existing efforts. The working group should also address standard reporting for other toxicological end-points.

2.2 Lipid-soluble residues of veterinary drugs with MRLs in milk

The Committee at its present meeting considered the potential public health impact of lipid-soluble residues of veterinary drugs in milk, in cases in which milk fat may be used for production of processed dairy products. Examples of classes of particular compounds include, but are not necessarily limited to, those such as the macrocyclic lactones and pyrethroids.

The Committee has routinely tried, where possible, to harmonize its recommendations on MRLs with those issued by JMPR and by the Codex Committee on Pesticide Residues (CCPR), particularly in situations in which a substance may be used as a pesticide or as a veterinary drug. For substances such as the cypermethrins, for example, JMPR recommends MRLs in animal milk on the basis of content of milk fat. In this regard, to report an MRL for a lipid-soluble compound in cows' milk on the basis of milk fat would be consistent with JMPR procedures. Furthermore, this would permit the Committee to consider recommending a single MRL for a substance, regardless of whether it was originally administered as a veterinary drug or as a pesticide.

At its previous meetings, when considering MRLs for these classes of compounds, the Committee has limited its recommendations to MRLs in fresh milk, rather than including recommendations for

MRLs in milk fat, where large concentration factors occur. This is consistent with the definition of an MRL in raw, unprocessed products. However, the definition does take into account other relevant risks, as well as aspects of food technology. The potential effect of reporting an MRL on the basis of milk fat is demonstrated by the example of a substance that has an MRL of 1 mg/kg in whole milk. If fresh milk is composed of 4% milk fat, the MRL in milk fat would be 25 mg/kg (1 mg/kg ÷ 0.04 = 25 mg/kg), assuming all residue partitions into the milk fat.

In situations where milk or milk fat is used to produce commodities such as butter and cheese, the finished product may contain a very high percentage of milk fat, and thus very large amounts of residues. These highly elevated amounts of residues in the finished, processed product may exceed an amount that might pose public health concerns, for example, that could result in amounts of residues that may exhibit a toxic effect in humans. Such a determination would have to be considered on a case-by-case basis.

Recognizing the potential public health consequences thus identified, the Committee requested early consideration by the Codex Committee on Residues of Veterinary Drugs (CCRVDF), in its role as risk manager, on how JECFA should proceed in the future in cases in which MRLs of lipid-soluble residues originating from the use of veterinary drugs are identified in milk. It should be noted that if CCRVDF indicated to the Committee that it should proceed in the manner described, it would be necessary for the Committee to reconsider its recommendations for MRLs for lipid-soluble residues in whole milk.

2.3 Statistical methods for the estimation of MRLs

At several of its previous meetings, the Committee decided that it is desirable to use statistical methods when deriving MRLs for veterinary drugs, whenever a suitable database is available. A statistical approach was taken on several occasions when the data met the necessary criteria.

This statistical approach included:

— Linear regression analysis of data describing the terminal depletion of a suitable marker residue in edible tissues following the (last) administration of the drug under approved conditions of use;
— Subsequent use of the results of the regression analysis for the estimation of upper limits of the 95% (alternatively, 99%) confi-

dence interval (CI) for the upper one-sided tolerance limit on the 95th (alternatively, 99th) percentile of the population sampled;

— Iterative calculation of statistical limits, such as a function of time over the whole phase of terminal elimination of the marker residue;

— The statistical method includes a mechanism for the derivation of MRLs for veterinary drugs from a set of data.

Since the necessary calculations are complex and should be performed reproducibly and in a fully transparent manner, the Secretariat supported the development of a tool that is based on spreadsheets and that facilitates the application of the necessary statistical tests to data on kinetic residue depletion and the calculation of the above-mentioned statistical tolerance limits. The currently available trial version supported the estimation of suitable MRLs for edible tissues. The workbook used only basic Microsoft Excel instructions. In order to allow the user to control each and every calculation and to fully understand the procedure, no sophisticated programming was used.

The Committee welcomed the initiative of the Secretariat and recommended that the Secretariat should continue with the necessary steps:

— To further improve the current applications and the documentation of the tool;

— To extend the applicability of the tool to include estimation of MRLs for milk;

— To publish the tool and invite all interested parties to comment on it;

— To test and validate the tool.

2.4 Terminology for analytical methods (from the Codex Committee on Methods of Analysis and Sampling)

The Committee considered a document (CL 2003/43-MAS) prepared by the Codex Committee on Methods of Analysis and Sampling (CCMAS), on proposed revisions to definitions of analytical terminology contained in the *Codex Alimentarius Commission, Procedural Manual*[2]). The Committee noted that the Committee's own report, FAO Food and Nutrition Paper No. 41/14, contains a section on *Requirements for Validation of Analytical Methods.* In general, the document prepared by CCMAS references Codex definitions and provides guidance on the experimental data required in response to

---

[2] *Codex Alimentarius Commission. Procedural Manual.* Thirteenth edition. Joint FAO/WHO Food Standards Programme, 2004.

the definitions. Several proposed revisions of these definitions, however, are of analytical terms that are also defined in the FAO Food and Nutrition Paper No. 41/14. The Committee was also aware that the Codex Committee on Residues of Veterinary Drugs in Foods (CCRVDF) was reviewing requirements for analytical methods for residues of veterinary drugs in foods. The Committee agreed in principle that definitions of analytical terminology used in documents published by the Committee should be harmonized with those used in the *Codex Alimentarius Commission Procedural Manual*, and in *Codex Alimentarius Vol. 3 — Residues of Veterinary Drugs in Foods*[3].

As work was in progress in the Codex Committees and final definitions had not been approved by the Codex Alimentarius Commission, the Committee at its present meeting agreed that this matter should be considered at its next meeting. The Committee also recommended that an expert should be assigned to review and report on the status of this matter at that meeting.

2.5 Response to the Codex Committee on Residues of Veterinary Drugs in Foods on its Draft Risk Assessment Policy

At its sixtieth meeting, the Committee had provided answers to CCRVDF on some specific questions regarding risk assessment principles[4]. At the request of FAO and WHO, the Committee at its present meeting reviewed Annex I of the *Discussion Paper on Risk Analysis Principles and Methodologies in the Codex Committee on Residue of Veterinary Drugs in Food*[5].

Although the Committee recognized the value of a risk assessment policy, it was concerned that the current draft document to CCRVDF was inadequate, because of serious flaws in its structure and content.

At its present meeting, the Committee agreed that Annex I of the above-mentioned draft discussion paper in its current form required substantial revision, which should address the following issues:

— A risk assessment policy should provide a general policy framework for the work of risk assessors and not describe the details of the four steps of the risk assessment process.
— The roles and responsibilities of risk assessors and risk managers need to be clearly defined, recognizing the independence and transparency of the risk assessment process.

---

[3] *Codex Alimentarius Vol. 3 — Residues of Veterinary Drugs in Foods*, Second Edition, 1996.
[4] ftp://ftp.fao.org/es/esn/jecfa/ccrvdf60.pdf
[5] Document CX/RVDF 01/9: ftp://ftp.fao.org/codex/ccrvdf13/rv01_09e.pdf

— The development of risk assessment guidelines is an inherent part of the corresponding scientific work that needs to be accomplished by risk assessors.
— The Expert Committee is an independent scientific body that provides advice not only to Codex but also directly to FAO and WHO and to Member countries. The risk assessment policy needs to recognize these related but independent roles of the Committee.
— The Committee noted that similar activities are ongoing in other Codex Committees (e.g. Codex Committee on Food Additives and Contaminants (CCFAC), Codex Committee on Food Hygiene (CCFH), Codex Committee on Pesticide Residues (CCPR)) and therefore strongly recommended that every effort be made to harmonize these activities.

The Committee recommended that a risk assessment policy (principles and processes) should include at least the following elements:

— Objectives of a risk assessment;
— Responsibilities of the risk manager and risk assessor in the process of problem formulation;
— Need and mechanisms for effective dialogue between risk manager and risk assessor;
— Core principles to conduct a risk assessment (e.g. scientific soundness, transparency, etc.);
— Inputs to the risk assessment (e.g. sources of data, confidentiality etc.);
— Outputs of the risk assessment (form and detail, including request for different risk management options and their consequences);
— Level of protection to be provided by the risk assessment.

The Committee welcomed the opportunity to comment on the current document; the Joint Secretariat was asked to continue discussion with CCRVDF and to consider the possibility that members of the Committee could be consulted in a written procedure before the next meeting of the Committee. The Committee suggested that close co-ordination with other ongoing activities was also desirable.

3. **Comments on residues of specific veterinary drugs**

The Committee considered one veterinary drug for the first time and re-evaluated nine others. Information on the safety evaluations is summarized in Annex 2. Details of further toxicological studies and other information required for certain substances are given in Annex 3.

3.1 Cefuroxime

Cefuroxime is a cephalosporin antibacterial agent that is active against a range of Gram-positive and Gram-negative bacteria. Intramammary infusions of cefuroxime are used in veterinary medicine for the treatment of clinical mastitis in lactating cattle and for dry-cow therapy. Cefuroxime is also used in human medicine.

At its fifty-eighth meeting (Annex 1, reference *157*), the Committee established a temporary ADI for cefuroxime of 0–30 µg/kg bw on the basis of the MIC_{50} for *Bifidobacterium* spp. The Committee also noted that a toxicological ADI of 0–4 mg/kg bw could be established on the basis of a no-observed-effect level (NOEL) for cefuroxime of 400 mg/kg bw per day for haematological changes identified in a 27-week study of toxicity in dogs treated orally, and applying a safety factor of 100.

The evaluation of cefuroxime residues performed by the Committee at its fifty-eighth meeting showed that a large percentage of the total radiolabelled residue in milk had not been identified. In pooled milk collected from eight cows, for example, >80% of the total radiolabelled residue was not identified in samples from the first, second, third and fifth milkings, corresponding to 12, 24, 36 and 60 h after the last treatment. The mean concentrations of total radiolabelled cefuroxime equivalents in these pooled samples were 270, 38, 16 and 2 mg/kg, respectively. The concentrations of total radiolabelled cefuroxime equivalents were <1 mg/kg at the sixth and subsequent milkings and <0.1 mg/kg at the tenth and subsequent milkings.

The Committee at its previous meetings has discounted the significance of unidentified residues that comprise ≤10% of the total residue, by considering them as equally potent as the parent compound. In the case of cefuroxime, the unidentified residues represented >80% of the total, thus justifying the need for a more complete identification of the toxicological significance of these residues.

Therefore, the Committee at its fifty-eighth meeting in 2002 requested that the following information be provided for evaluation in 2004: the results of studies to (1) identify the residues in milk and clarify whether the residues other than parent compound are due primarily to metabolism or to non-metabolic decomposition of cefuroxime; and (2) characterize the toxicological significance of non-parent radiolabelled residues in milk.

No new data were supplied for review by the present Committee. Instead, the sponsor provided an expert report that included a re-evaluation of previously submitted data. To address the questions posed by the Committee at its fifty-eighth meeting, the report explained that:

— Given the emphasis of the Committee on the antimicrobial activity of cefuroxime residues, the characterization of residues devoid of antimicrobial activity was perceived as not important. Therefore, no attempt had been made to characterize the toxicological importance of unidentified residues.
— Identification of the unidentified fraction of the total radiolabelled residue might have been feasible in milk collected up to the third milking after the last treatment, when concentrations of all residues were at their highest levels, but this was not done and the samples had since been destroyed.
— After the fifth milking, when the concentration of cefuroxime would be in compliance with the MRL, the identification of transformation products would have been impossible, owing to the small amount of radiolabelled residue present at this time and the poor resolution of components by radio-analysis and high-performance liquid chromatography (HPLC).
— The appearance of unidentified cefuroxime residues was not caused by species differences in metabolism but by the route of administration. Metabolites may not have been detected in studies of pharmacokinetics in healthy animals or humans, owing to the rapid clearance of cefuroxime from plasma. Therefore, it was reasoned that cefuroxime infused into the udder could be metabolized during the 12 h between milkings. However, it could not be determined with any degree of certainty whether the unidentified residue fraction consisted of the products of metabolism or of non-metabolic degradation.
— The toxicological profile of the unidentified residue remains unknown.

The Committee noted that the sponsor's expert report also drew attention to the observation that cefuroxime is poorly absorbed from the udder and therefore consumer exposure to tissue residues would be minimal. This was supported by the conclusions of the Committee at its fifty-eighth meeting after review of a residue study in dairy cows treated with cefuroxime by intramammary infusion. Seven days after administration of cefuroxime, total concentrations of radiolabelled residues in tissues had declined to near or below the limits of detection. The present Committee also noted that unidentified radiolabelled residues were also detected in kidney tissue.

The Committee re-evaluated the residue depletion study submitted by the sponsor and noted that when milk samples were re-analysed by high-performance liquid chromatography–mass spectrometry (HPLC–MS), 14 days after the first analysis, significantly lower concentrations of cefuroxime were measured in all samples. The Committee posed additional technical questions to the manufacturer in relation to milk sample collection, storage, and cefuroxime stability in milk samples that had been frozen and thawed before analysis. On the basis of the answers provided, the Committee concluded that it was unable to confirm the ratio of cefuroxime to cefuroxime-related residues identified at the fifty-eighth meeting. The Committee further concluded that data from this study could not be further considered for the purpose of establishing an MRL for cefuroxime in cows' milk.

The present Committee also considered the results of studies reported in the published literature, which show that cefuroxime is unstable in aqueous solutions, including biological matrices, at temperatures >30 °C. Descarbamoyl cefuroxime, a degradation product of the hydrolysis of cefuroxime, and other products of hydrolysis have been identified in various studies.

On the basis of this information, the Committee concluded that it is likely that cefuroxime is unstable in the udder environment and also in milk samples subjected to repeated freeze–thaw cycles. It cannot be determined from the currently available information whether unidentified cefuroxime residues in milk are products of metabolism or of simple degradation.

The Committee reviewed published studies on the pharmacokinetics of cefuroxime in human patients with renal insufficiency and thus decreased clearance of cefuroxime from plasma. Metabolism of cefuroxime was not observed in these patients. Therefore, the Committee concluded that the data did not support the sponsor's suggestion that increased metabolism of cefuroxime may occur after longer periods of systemic exposure.

Evaluation
After consideration of all available data, including additional residue information provided to the Committee and considering that:

— No new information had been provided in response to requests for data on the identification and toxicity of the unidentified residues of cefuroxime in milk;
— The Committee was unable to adequately evaluate the metabolism or degradation of cefuroxime in milk; and

— The radiolabelled-residue depletion study in cows could no longer be used to determine the relationship between residues of parent compound, other antimicrobial active residues and total residues of cefuroxime.

The present Committee concluded that it could not extend the temporary ADI or MRLs established at its fifty-eighth meeting. Therefore, the temporary ADI and MRLs for cefuroxime in milk were not extended and therefore withdrawn.

Addenda to the toxicological monograph and the residue evaluation were prepared.

3.2 Cyhalothrin

Cyhalothrin is a type II pyrethroid insecticide and acaricide that is used predominantly on cattle and sheep, and to a lesser extent on pigs and goats, for the control of a broad range of ectoparasites.

The Committee evaluated cyhalothrin at its fifty-fourth meeting (Annex 1, reference *146*), when it established a temporary ADI of 0–0.002 mg/kg bw by applying a safety factor of 500 to the lowest-observed-effect level (LOEL) of 1 mg/kg bw per day for induction of liquid faeces in dogs in a 26-week study. The high safety factor was used to compensate for the absence of a NOEL in this study. The ADI was designated as temporary because the Committee was concerned that neurobehavioural effects had not been adequately investigated. In order to enable a full ADI to be established, the Committee at its fifty-fourth meeting required the results of studies appropriate for identifying a NOEL for neurobehavioural effects in laboratory animals, to be submitted for evaluation in 2002.

The Committee reconsidered the toxicological data on cyhalothrin at its fifty-eighth meeting in 2002 (Annex 1, reference *157*) and decided to extend the temporary ADI while awaiting the results of a study of neurobehaviour. These data were required for evaluation in 2004.

Toxicological data
The present Committee considered the results of a new study of neurobehavioural effects with cyhalothrin and of two new reports of tests for genotoxicity with lambda-cyhalothrin (λ-cyhalothrin), which is the most active of the isomer pairs in cyhalothrin.

The Committee at its fifty-fourth meeting had considered data on the genotoxicity of cyhalothrin and λ-cyhalothrin and concluded that cyhalothrin appeared to be non-genotoxic. A range of studies of genotoxicity (tests for reverse mutation in bacteria, cell transformation in vitro, cytogenetic effects in the bone marrow of rats treated in vivo, and for dominant lethal mutation in mice) had given uniformly negative results. A more extensive range of tests for genotoxicity had been performed on λ-cyhalothrin, with most of them giving negative results (tests for reverse mutation in bacteria, gene mutation in mammalian cells in vitro, unscheduled DNA synthesis in vitro, cytogenetic effects in vitro, and for micronucleus formation in mice in vivo). A test for micronucleus formation in fish had given a positive result, but this was disregarded, as the relevance to human health of a positive result in this assay was not known.

One of the new studies of genotoxicity considered by the present Committee was a test for micronucleus formation in fish. Although λ-cyhalothrin gave positive results in this test, it was noted by the Committee that this assay was not validated for use in human risk assessment and again the positive result was disregarded, as the relevance to human health was not known.

A new report described an assay for cytogenetic effects in the bone marrow of rats treated *in vivo*. Increased incidences of chromosomal aberrations in bone marrow cells and of micronuclei in polychromatic erythrocytes indicated that λ-cyhalothrin was genotoxic under the conditions of the assay. It was noted by the Committee that the protocols of these assays in the bone marrow of rats deviated from internationally-agreed methodological guidelines in that small group sizes, extended periods of dosing and late harvest times were used. These deviations could make the tests oversensitive and unreliable. The positive result reported for λ-cyhalothrin in the new assay for cytogenetic effects in the bone marrow of rats in vivo was considered in the context of the tests for genotoxicity that had been evaluated at earlier meetings. Considering the negative results of earlier, well-conducted tests with cyhalothrin and λ-cyhalothrin in vivo to be more reliable than the positive results of the new study, the Committee concluded that the data as a whole suggested that cyhalothrin presents no genotoxic hazard to humans.

The results of a new series of experiments in rats on the neurobehavioural effects of cyhalothrin administered orally for 7 days indicated a NOEL of 1.0 mg/kg bw per day, with various behavioural changes and increased serum corticosterone concentrations being observed at a dose of 3 mg/kg bw per day. The Committee noted that the NOEL for this study was the lowest NOEL for toxicological effects in rats and was numerically the same as the LOEL for liquid faeces in dogs, which had been used to set the temporary ADI for cyhalothrin.

Comparison of the results of the studies of toxicity in rats with those in dogs suggested that cyhalothrin is of similar toxicity in the two species. The Committee decided that the temporary ADI could be replaced by an ADI of 0–0.005 mg/kg bw, which was determined by dividing the LOEL of 1 mg/kg bw per day for dogs (also the NOEL for rats) by a safety factor of 200. The safety factor incorporated a factor of 2 to compensate for the absence of a NOEL for dogs. An additional factor was considered appropriate because: liquid faeces is a common minor health effect in dogs, and some liquid faeces also occurred in control dogs; the LOEL was close to a NOEL; and because there was a clear NOEL for neurobehavioural effects in rats.

An addendum to the toxicological monograph was prepared.

3.3 Cypermethrin and α-cypermethrin

Cypermethrin and α-cypermethrin are highly active pyrethroid insecticides, which are effective in public health and animal husbandry, and against a wide range of pests in agriculture. Cypermethrin has been widely used throughout the world since the late 1970s, while α-cypermethrin has been available commercially since the mid 1980s. The present Committee responded to a request from CCRVDF at its Fourteenth Session (*2*) to consider the establishment of a common ADI and common MRLs, for both cypermethrin and α-cypermethrin.

At its forty-seventh meeting (Annex 1, reference *125*), the Committee evaluated cypermethrin and α-cypermethrin and established an ADI of 0–0.05 mg/kg bw for cypermethrin and 0–0.02 mg/kg bw for α-cypermethrin. The Joint FAO/WHO Meeting on Pesticide Residues (JMPR) had also evaluated cypermethrin and established an ADI of 0–0.05 mg/kg bw (*3, 4*).

The Committee at its fifty-eighth meeting recommended the following MRLs, expressed as cypermethrin, for sheep tissues: 20 µg/kg in muscle, liver and kidney, and 200 µg/kg in fat. MRLs for fat were based on residue studies using a pour-on formulation, reported at the fifty-fourth meeting. The MRLs in muscle, liver and kidney recommended were based upon twice the limit of quantitation of the method (10 µg/kg).

The MRLs, expressed as α-cypermethrin, for cattle and sheep tissues and cows' milk, that were recommended by the Committee at its fifty-eighth meeting were: muscle, liver and kidney, 100 µg/kg; fat, 1000 µg/kg and cows' milk, 100 µg/kg. MRLs in fat, muscle and cows' milk were based on residue data of studies submitted for evaluation. MRLs in liver and kidney were recommended based on twice the limit of quantification of the methods used (LOQ = 20 µg/kg for sheep tissues, 50 µg/kg for cattle tissues).

Cypermethrin typically contains 20–40% α-cypermethrin. The Committee noted that α-cypermethrin comprises the two most toxicologically active isomers of cypermethrin. As the ratio of isomers in commercial cypermethrin products is variable, the toxicity of these products also varies. The NOEL for α-cypermethrin alone was lower than that for cypermethrin. However, the observed toxicity was qualitatively similar. The Committee also noted that the metabolism of α-cypermethrin and of cypermethrin is similar, although not identical.

At its present meeting, the Committee received only new data on analytical methods.

Evaluation

The Committee concluded that as α-cypermethrin alone and cypermethrin are qualitatively similar in their toxicity and metabolism, and in view of the fact that cypermethrin includes a substantial proportion of α-cypermethrin, the ADI previously established for α-cypermethrin could apply for both substances. α-Cypermethrin is more toxic than cypermethrin, and the proportion of α-cypermethrin in cypermethrin may depend on the commercial source. The Committee reconfirmed the NOEL for α-cypermethrin of 1.5 mg/kg bw per day on the basis of a 52-week study in dogs fed with α-cypermethrin, as identified at the forty-seventh meeting.

The Committee established a group ADI of 0–0.02 mg/kg bw for cypermethrin and α-cypermethrin, using a safety factor of 100 and by rounding up.

Residue data

No new residue depletion studies were presented to the sixty-second meeting of the Committee. Studies provided to the fifty-eighth meeting of the Committee indicated that, in cattle treated with a formulation of [^{14}C]α-cypermethrin at a dose of 3 mg/kg, maximum concentrations of α-cypermethrin residues were: back fat, 647 µg/kg; omental fat, 421 µg/kg, kidney, 22 µg/kg, muscle, 35 µg/kg; and liver, <30 µg/kg analysed either by HPLC using a radiolabel detector or by gas chromatography–electron capture detector (GC–ECD). Maximum concentrations of α-cypermethrin residues in sheep treated with a topical dose of 15 mg/kg were: 1323 µg/kg for back fat; 314 µg/kg for omental fat; 22 µg/kg for kidney; and <20 µg/kg for muscle and liver. In milk, the highest concentration of residues found was 89 µg/kg at 60 h after the last treatment. The highest concentration of residues found in fat of sheep treated topically at the recommended dose was

34 µg/kg, while residues in liver, muscle and kidney were below the LOQ (10 µg/kg) of the GC–ECD method used.

Analytical methods

Three analytical GC–ECD methods used for the determination of cypermethrin residues in cattle and sheep tissues and in cows' milk were submitted to the Committee at its present meeting. The methods are almost identical and are suitable for determining the concentrations of cypermethrin residues in cattle and sheep tissues and cows' milk over a range of 10 to 400 µg/kg. For cattle and sheep tissues, the LOQs were 100 µg/kg for fat and 10 µg/kg for liver, muscle and kidney. The LOQ was 10 µg/kg for cows' milk.

Maximum residue limits

In recommending a suitable marker residue and common MRLs for cypermethrins used as veterinary drugs, the Committee considered the following factors:

— α-Cypermethrin consists of two of the four *cis* isomers present in cypermethrin.
— A group ADI for α-cypermethrin and cypermethrin of 0–0.02 mg/kg bw, which is equivalent to 0–1200 µg per day for a 60 kg person, was established for the most toxicologically active substance (α-cypermethrin).
— Using the common analytical methods for residue control, the eight isomers of cypermethrin cannot be resolved and a single, fused chromatographic peak is obtained. Therefore, residues reported represent the sum of all isomers.

After considering the request for a common set of recommendations for residues of cypermethrin and α-cypermethrin in cattle and sheep tissues and rounding, as appropriate, the Committee recommended the following MRLs, expressed as the total of cypermethrin residues: muscle, liver and kidney, 50 µg/kg; fat, 1000 µg/kg; and milk, 100 µg/kg. The recommended MRLs in muscle, liver and kidney were based on the limits of quantitation of the new methods, considering that the concentration of residues in both cattle and sheep tissues was ≤35 µg/kg. The MRLs for fat and cows' milk were based on residue depletion data. These MRLs replace those previously recommended.

Residues in cattle tissues are lower than those in sheep tissues, according to studies using the maximum permitted dose of α-cypermethrin; therefore, the same MRLs apply to both species.

Using the daily food consumption factors, these recommended MRLs would result in a theoretical maximum daily intake of 368 µg of residues as cypermethrin equivalents, or 30% of the upper bound of the ADI for a 60 kg person. The exposure to cypermethrin from use of pesticides, as estimated by JMPR, is approximately 300 µg. The total theoretical exposure for the cypermethrins would therefore be approximately 650 µg.

The Committee recommended that JMPR should also consider this approach.

3.4 Doramectin

Doramectin is an ecto- and endoparasiticide for use in cattle and pigs. It is a semisynthetic member of the avermectin class, and is structurally similar to abamectin and ivermectin. Doramectin was first reviewed by the Committee at its forty-fifth meeting (Annex 1, reference *119*) when an ADI of 0–0.5 µg/kg bw was established and the following MRLs were recommended, for cattle: muscle, 10 µg/kg; liver, 100 µg/kg; kidney, 30 µg/kg; and fat, 150 µg/kg, expressed as parent drug. Applying these MRLs, the theoretical maximum daily intake was 33 µg per day. The Committee at its fifty-eighth meeting (Annex 1, reference *157*) concluded that the additional safety factor of 2 used to establish the ADI by the Committee at its forty-fifth meeting was no longer necessary and established an ADI for doramectin of 0–1 µg/kg bw.

The Fourteenth Session of CCRVDF (*2*) requested consideration of a MRL for cows' milk. The sponsor submitted three new residue depletion studies for doramectin, to extend its use to lactating cattle for the control of internal and external parasites. The recommended pour-on dose is 0.5 mg/kg bw, while the injectable dose is 0.2 mg/kg bw. At the present meeting, two studies using the pour-on formulation and one using the injectable formulation were reviewed. In addition, performance data were provided for the analytical method to determine residues of doramectin in milk from lactating dairy cattle.

Milk residue studies
In the first study, 10 dairy Holstein cows were treated with a pour-on formulation of doramectin at a dose of 0.58 mg/kg bw and were retreated with the same dose 56 days later. The study was conducted according to good laboratory practice (GLP). Samples of milk were collected for 49 days and 10 days, respectively, after the first and second treatments. Samples were collected twice daily until day 7, and once daily on days 10, 13, 16, 19, 22, 25, 28, 32, 36, 40 and 49. On retreatment, samples were taken twice daily until day 7 and once at day 10. The analyses of doramectin milk residue and milk/fat residue were

performed using a validated HPLC and fluorescence detector method.

In the same study, the concentrations of doramectin residue in milk increased to a maximum mean value of 22 μg/kg at 72 h after treatment. Mean concentrations of doramectin residues decreased to below the limit of quantitation (3 μg/kg) at 384 h (16 days). After re-treatment, concentrations of doramectin residues increased gradually to a maximum mean value of 12 μg/kg at 48 h after dosing; and decreased to <4 μg/kg at 240 h (10 days) after dosing. The milk/fat analyses were conducted 1, 4, and 10 days after dosing. Mean concentrations of doramectin residues in the milk fat at these time points were 171 μg/kg, 501 μg/kg and 114 μg/kg, respectively. Concentration factors for doramectin residues in milk fat were 29.6, 32.2 and 24.7, respectively.

In the second study, 10 cows were treated with doramectin by topical application of a pour-on formulation at a dose of 0.58 mg/kg and were re-treated with the same dose 56 days later. Samples of milk were collected twice daily. Concentrations of doramectin in milk increased to a maximum mean value of 9 μg/kg at 45 h after treatment and decreased to below the LOQ by 237 h (10 days) after treatment. After re-treatment on day 56, concentrations of residues increased to a mean maximum value of 8 μg/kg after 93 h and decreased to less than the LOQ after 237 h (10 days). Mean concentrations of doramectin residues in the milk fat at 1, 4, and 10 days were 91 μg/kg, 142 μg/kg and 55 μg/kg, respectively. Concentration factors for doramectin residues in milk fat versus milk were 14.2, 20.9 and 14.1, respectively.

Differences in residue concentrations between the two studies with pour-on doramectin were attributed to climatic and production factors.

The third study determined the residue depletion profile of doramectin following the subcutaneous administration of doramectin formulation at 0.23 mg/kg bw in lactating cattle, followed by re-treatment at the same dose 56 days later. Sampling followed the same protocol as the two previous studies. The analysis of doramectin milk residues was conducted using the HPLC–fluorescence detection method noted previously. Doramectin concentrations in milk increased gradually to a maximum mean value of 45 μg/kg at 67 h. Subsequently, doramectin residues gradually declined, with mean residues below LOQ at 523 h (22 days). After re-treatment, doramectin residues increased to a maximum mean value of 53 μg/kg at 56 h. Residue concentrations then decreased to a mean value of 25 μg/kg at 237 h (10 days) after re-treatment. Residues resulting from treatment by injection were consistently higher at any given time-point than were those resulting from treatment with the pour-on formulation. Milk fat analyses were conducted using samples collected at the morning milking on days 1, day 4 and day 10 after treatment. Mean concentrations of doramectin residues in milk fat at these time-points were 557 µg/kg, 1036 µg/kg and 354 µg/kg, respectively. Milk fat concentration factors were 24, 24.2 and 23.4, respectively.

Analytical methods
A study was conducted to validate analytical methodology for the recovery and quantitation of doramectin residues in cows' milk. In the method validation, aliquots of milk were fortified with doramectin and the internal standard and were extracted before analysis by HPLC–fluorescence. The method is based on the extraction procedure used for tissue and requires on-column conversion to a fluorescence derivative. The limit of quantification was set at 3 µg/kg. The recovery estimated at the LOQ was 95%. Method performance data indicate that it is suitable for use in residue depletion studies and for routine surveillance purposes.

Maximum residue limits
In recommending MRLs for doramectin in milk, the Committee considered the following factors:

— The ADI for doramectin was 0–1 µg/kg bw, equivalent to an intake of up to 60 µg per day for a 60 kg person
— Based on MRLs for tissues in cattle and pigs, and the theoretical maximum daily intake of residues in tissue of 33 µg per day, approximately 27 µg per day are available for milk.
— Based on its limited metabolism and the known large partitioning ratio for residues between milk fat and aqueous milk, the Committee considers that the ratio for marker residue to total residue for doramectin in milk would be equivalent to the ratio of doramectin residues in fat (0.80).
— The residue studies provided used a pour-on formulation at 0.58 mg/kg bw and the injectable formulation at 0.23 mg/kg, somewhat in excess of the recommended doses of 0.5 mg/kg bw and 0.2 mg/kg bw, respectively.
— The marker residue is doramectin.
— A suitable analytical method is available for determining residues in milk.

Based on the factors noted above, the Committee considered recommending an MRL on the basis of the available portion of doramectin residues permitted by the ADI. The Committee recommended an MRL of 15 µg/kg, determined as doramectin. Taking into account the marker residue to total residue ratio in fat (0.8) and 1.5 kg of milk in the model food diet, this would be equivalent to 28 µg. Total residues of doramectin for muscle, liver, kidney and fat tissues and cows' milk, estimated from the model food diet, would be 61 µg/kg.

The Committee noted that on the basis of an MRL of 15 µg/kg for doramectin in whole milk in cattle, the milk discard times would be approximately 240 h according to the studies using the pour-on treatment. Milk discard times would be approximately 480 h after treatment using the dose formulated for injection. The Committee noted that in milk containing 4% milk fat, the residues in milk fat would be equivalent to 375 µg/kg (15 µg/kg ÷ 0.04 = 375 µg/kg). This is higher than the MRL of 150 µg/kg in fat tissue.

The Committee noted that the discard time necessary to accommodate the recommended MRL in milk was unlikely to be consistent with good veterinary practice.

An addendum to the residue evaluation was prepared.

3.5 Flumequine

Flumequine is a fluoroquinolone compound with antimicrobial activity against Gram-negative organisms and is used in the treatment of enteric infections in food animals. It also has limited use in humans for the treatment of urinary-tract infections. Flumequine was evaluated by the Committee at its forty-second, forty-eighth, fifty-fourth and sixtieth meetings (Annex 1, references *110*, *128*, *146* and *162*). At its forty-eighth meeting, the Committee established an ADI of 0–30 µg/kg bw on the basis of hepatotoxicity in male CD-1 mice in a 13-week study. The Committee at that meeting concluded that flumequine was considered to be a non-genotoxic hepatocarcinogen, and that the induction of hepatocellular necrosis-regeneration cycles by hepatotoxicity was considered to be the relevant mechanism for induction of liver tumours in mice.

At its sixtieth meeting, the Committee evaluated new studies that had been carried out to further elucidate the mechanism of flumequine-induced hepatocarcinogenicity in mice. On the basis of these new studies, the Committee could not dismiss the possibility that flumequine induces tumours in the mouse liver by a mechanism that includes genotoxic effects. The Committee therefore concluded that it could not support an ADI and withdrew the ADI that had been established at its forty-eighth meeting. The Committee expressed the wish to receive additional data on the mechanism involved in tumour formation before re-establishment of an ADI could be considered. The present Committee evaluated a new study investigating the genotoxic potential of flumequine in a test for unscheduled DNA synthesis in the liver in vivo.

Toxicological data

In short-term and long-term studies of toxicity that were evaluated by the Committee at its forty-second and forty-eighth meetings, oral administration of flumequine caused dose-related hepatotoxic effects in rats and CD-1 mice. The liver damage was most pronounced in male mice, and included degenerative changes with hypertrophy, fatty vacuolation, focal necrosis and increased mitotic activity. After cessation of treatment with flumequine, the liver damage was reversed. Treatment with flumequine had little or no effect on P450-dependent hepatic drug-metabolizing enzymes or on glucuronyl transferase. Flumequine increased the plasma activities of alanine and aspartate aminotransferases, alkaline phosphatase and lactate dehydrogenase. The overall NOEL for hepatotoxic effects in mice was 25 mg/kg bw per day.

The results of long-term studies of toxicity that were evaluated by the Committee at its forty-second meeting showed that flumequine had no carcinogenic effects in rats, whereas in CD-1 mice an increase in the incidence of liver tumours was observed at oral doses of flumequine of ≥400 mg/kg bw per day (the lowest dose tested) in an 18-month study. The incidence of tumours in male mice was significantly higher than that in female mice. In male mice, the incidence of liver tumours increased in a dose-related and time-dependent manner, and was paralleled by an increase in the incidence of hepatotoxic changes.

The present Committee re-evaluated the three short-term studies that used a two-stage hepatocarcinogenesis protocol in mice. In these studies, which were presented to the Committee at its sixtieth meeting, treatment with flumequine caused the development of basophilic liver foci, which could suggest that flumequine has tumour-initiating potential. The Committee also noted, however, that concurrent hepatotoxicity (evidenced by pale, vacuolated hepatocytes with fatty droplets, inflammatory cell infiltration, increased mitotic figures and/or necrosis) was observed, and a regenerative response to these toxic changes and indications of oxidative stress.

Flumequine gave negative results in various assays for genotoxicity that were evaluated by the Committee at its forty-second meeting. These included assays in vitro in bacteria (reverse mutation in

Salmonella typhimurium) and mammalian cells (gene mutation at the *Hprt* locus in lymphoma cells in mice and gene mutation in Chinese hamster ovary cells), and an assay for chromosome aberration in rat bone marrow in vivo. At its sixtieth meeting, the Committee evaluated a comet assay in which flumequine sporadically caused DNA strand breaks in the liver in vivo. Although this could indicate that flumequine has genotoxic activity, the Committee also noted the limitations of this assay and that the effect in the liver was only marginal.

The Committee at its present meeting also evaluated a new, adequately conducted test for unscheduled DNA synthesis with flumequine in rat liver cells in vivo. The result of this test was negative, indicating that flumequine does not interact directly with liver DNA.

Evaluation
The Committee concluded that the available data support a non-genotoxic, threshold-based mechanism for tumour formation by flumequine in the mouse liver. The Committee therefore re-established the ADI of 0–30 µg/kg bw that it had originally established for flumequine at its forty-eighth meeting. This ADI was based on the overall NOEL for hepatotoxicity of 25 mg/kg bw per day, observed in a 13-week study in mice, and a safety factor of 1000. A safety factor of 1000 was chosen to reflect the short duration of the study and the lack of histochemical characterization of the foci of altered hepatocytes.

Maximum residue limits
In view of its decision to re-establish the ADI for flumequine, the present Committee also agreed to re-establish the MRLs that had been established at its fifty-fourth meeting and withdrawn at its sixtieth meeting. For tissues from cattle, pig, sheep and chickens, the MRLs were: 500 µg/kg for muscle and liver; 3000 µg/kg for kidney; and 1000 µg/kg for fat. For trout muscle including normal proportions of skin, the MRL was 500 µg/kg.

The Committee recommended a temporary MRL of 500 µg/kg for muscle of black tiger shrimp (*Penaeus monodon*) on the basis of the evaluation made at its sixtieth meeting. The present Committee confirmed its previous request for the following information, to be submitted by 2006:

— A detailed description of a regulatory method, including its performance characteristics and validation data; and
— Information on the approved dose for treatment of black tiger shrimp and the results of residue depletion studies conducted at the recommended dose.

An addendum to the toxicological monograph was prepared.

3.6 Lincomycin

Lincomycin is a lincosamide antibiotic produced by *Streptomyces lincolnensis*. It is used alone or in combination with other drugs in poultry and pigs for oral treatment of bacterial enteric infections, control of respiratory infections and growth enhancement. Preparations of lincomycin administered by intramuscular injection are available for the treatment of bacterial enteric and respiratory disease in calves. Combination preparations of lincomycin and neomycin administered by intramammary infusion are used for treatment of mastitis in lactating dairy cattle.

Lincomycin was previously evaluated by the Committee at its fifty-fourth and fifty-eighth meetings (Annex 1, references *146* and *157*). At its fifty-fourth meeting, the Committee established an ADI of 0–30 µg/kg bw. The following temporary MRLs for cattle tissues were recommended: muscle, 100 µg/kg; liver, 500 µg/kg; kidney, 1500 µg/kg; and fat, 100 µg/kg. The MRL recommended for milk was 150 µg/kg.

The Committee at its fifty-fourth meeting requested data from residue depletion studies in cattle in order to confirm that lincomycin is the major microbiologically active residue in edible tissues. Since the requested data were not submitted at the fifty-eighth meeting, the temporary MRLs recommended by the Committee at its fifty-fourth meeting were withdrawn.

A new request to recommend MRLs for cattle was received from CCRVDF. The sponsor submitted data from four studies for consideration by the Committee; of these studies, three had been evaluated previously.

In the new study, 17 non-ruminating calves were given lincomycin by intramuscular administration at a dose of 10 mg/kg bw per day, given as two half doses on the first day of treatment, followed by a dose of 5 mg/kg bw per day for four consecutive days. Groups of animals were slaughtered on day 1, 7, 14, 21 or 28 after the last treatment. Samples of liver, kidney, muscle, fat and injection site were assayed for lincomycin residues using a microbiological method with a limit of detection of 0.1 mg/kg. Lincomycin was detected only in the liver (0.56 mg/kg), kidney (0.34 mg/kg) and injection site (0.26 mg/kg) at sampling on day 1. Lincomycin was not detected in any tissue 7 days after the last dose was administered.

Maximum residue limits

The Committee reviewed data from the new study and took into consideration the studies that it had evaluated at the fifty-fourth meeting. The data from these studies were considered insufficient to allow any extrapolation of the relationship between dose and residue concentration. In addition, the data from studies in non-ruminating calves could not be used to support a MRL for cows' milk.

Studies in pigs and chickens have shown significant differences between animal species in the kinetics of lincomycin residues in tissues. In pigs, concentrations of lincomycin residues in kidney were three times higher than those in liver, while in chickens the concentrations of residues in liver and kidney were similar. Therefore, the Committee concluded it was not possible to extrapolate the kinetics of lincomycin residues between species.

Since the available information was inadequate, the present Committee could not recommend MRLs for lincomycin in cattle tissues.

3.7 Melengestrol acetate

Melengestrol acetate (MGA) is a progestogen that is used as an animal feed additive to improve feed efficiency, increase the rate of body-weight gain, and suppress estrus in beef heifers. MGA is given at doses of 0.25–0.50 mg per heifer for 90–150 days before slaughter. The Committee at its fifty-fourth meeting (Annex 1, reference *146*) recommended temporary MRLs for cattle of 5 µg/kg in fat and 2 µg/kg in liver, and requested information on an analytical method suitable for the quantification of residues of MGA in liver and fat tissue. At its fifty-eighth meeting (Annex 1, reference *157*), the Committee concluded that the analytical method submitted for evaluation had been validated for monitoring compliance with the MRLs, and recommended that the temporary MRLs for cattle liver and fat be made permanent.

At its fifty-fourth meeting, the Committee was provided with insufficient information to characterize the structure and activity of the metabolites of MGA. When elaborating temporary MRLs, the Committee therefore assumed that the metabolites were equipotent to MGA in terms of progestogenic activity. New information regarding the structure and activity of the metabolites of MGA was submitted to the Committee for evaluation at its sixty-second meeting. Data on the metabolism of MGA in vitro, which provided the structural identities of the major metabolites of MGA, and a report describing the results of assays for transcriptional activation/reporter gene expression in vitro, which were used to determine the relative hormonal activities of MGA and its metabolites, were evaluated.

Metabolism
The extensive metabolism of MGA in several animal species and in humans was documented in previous reports. In the present studies,

the metabolic profile of MGA was characterized by means of the generation and isolation of metabolites in test systems in vitro, since the concentrations of metabolites in tissues and excreta from cattle fed with MGA were too low for this purpose. The test systems investigated used hepatic microsomes, hepatic $9000 \times g$ supernatant (S9), and liver slices, all of which were prepared from beef heifers. The metabolites were separated by semi-preparative HPLC and their structures were characterized by HPLC, HPLC–MS and nuclear magnetic resonance (NMR). Three monohydroxy metabolites, one dihydroxy metabolite, and several trace metabolites were generated in bovine hepatic microsomes. These metabolites were, in descending order of abundance: 2β-hydroxy-MGA (metabolite E), 6-hydroxymethyl-MGA (metabolite C), 15β-hydroxy-MGA (metabolite D), and 2β,15β-dihydroxy-MGA (metabolite B). Since metabolite A was generated only in trace amounts, its structure could not be determined. Additional metabolites formed in trace amounts by bovine hepatic microsomal systems were identified as monohydroxy and dihydroxy products. No conjugation products or additional metabolites of MGA were observed in bovine liver slices or bovine liver S9 fractions.

Rat microsomes, human microsomes and human recombinant cytochrome P450 generated metabolites B, C, D, and E, and additional minor metabolites. The latter were identified as monohydroxy and dihydroxy products; however, there were insufficient amounts for complete structure elucidation. The metabolism of MGA by human cytochrome P450 was shown to be primarily attributable to the CYP3A4 enzyme.

Steroid receptor specificity and relative potency of MGA metabolites
The small quantities of metabolites of MGA produced in cattle and in test systems in vitro were insufficient studies of efficacy or toxicology to be performed in either cattle or laboratory animal models in vivo. Therefore, the relative biological activity of MGA and its metabolites as agonists for the human progesterone receptor (PR) B-subtype, human glucocorticoid receptor (GR), human androgen receptor (AR), and human estrogen receptor α-subtype (ERα) was determined in assays for cell receptor activation and gene expression in vitro.

Samples of MGA, melengestrol, and metabolites B, C, D, and E were prepared. The purity of each metabolite was >95% by HPLC–UV. Comparator compounds for the PR assays (progesterone, a synthetic progestin R5020 and medroxyprogesterone acetate), the GR assays (dexamethasone, hydrocortisone and medroxyprogesterone acetate), the AR assays (dihydrotestosterone, a synthetic androgen R1881, progesterone and medroxyprogesterone acetate) and the ERα assays (17β-estradiol, ethinyl estradiol and medroxyprogesterone acetate) were also studied. Monkey kidney CV-1 cells were transiently co-transfected with the designated human steroid receptor expression vector and a luciferase reporter vector containing the appropriate hormone response element. The mouse mammary tumour virus–luciferase reporter vector (MMTV–Luc), which contains response elements for PR, GR, and AR was used for PR, GR, and AR assays, while the estrogen response element–luciferase reporter vector (ERE–Luc) was used for ERα assays. From the results of these assays, it was concluded that MGA and its metabolites exert their biological action primarily as progestogens and secondarily as gluco-corticoids. At relevant physiological concentrations, no activity was demonstrated in either the AR or ERα assays.

The bioactivity or potency (mg/kg of dose resulting in equal pharma-cological effect) of each compound relative to that of MGA was determined. Metabolite E was shown to be the most potent of the metabolites. The relative progestogenic activities of metabolite E and MGA were compared by fitting a concentration–effect curve to all the data. The concentration–effect curves for MGA and metabolite E were parallel. The predicted concentrations of MGA and metabolite E required to induce a response of 10%, 50% or 90% of the maximum were determined. The potency of metabolite E relative to MGA was 12.2% at the 10% induction level, 12.0% at the 50% induction level, and 11.8% at the 90% induction level.

Residue data
At its fifty-fourth meeting, the Committee noted that MGA, which is the marker residue, accounted for 33% of the total residues in liver and 85% of the total residues in fat in cattle. Moreover, the ratio of MGA in total residues, which was used to establish the MRLs for fat and liver, was based upon studies of the metabolism of the radiola-belled residue in animals slaughtered under conditions consistent with withdrawal on day 0 (6h after the last dose). The ratio of MGA residues in fat versus liver was 1.6:1. On the basis of the new informa-tion, the toxicological significance of the metabolites of MGA in tissue residues was considered further. Metabolite E, the most active me-tabolite, demonstrated, on average, 12% of the progestogenic potency of MGA, i.e. in order to achieve the same progestogenic activity as MGA, the dose of metabolite E given was, on average, 8.8-fold higher than that of MGA. The relative potency of metabolite E was then used to define the biological activity of the entire non-MGA fraction of the tissue residue, which potentially may be present in food for human consumption. This is a conservative

estimate since the activities of the other metabolites (B, C and D) were negligible, ranging from 0.09% to 0.23% that of MGA. On the basis of the relative potency of metabolite E, the non-MGA residues (fat, 15%; liver, 67%) were converted to MGA equivalents by reducing the percentage of MGA residues by 8.8-fold. This resulted in total MGA equivalents of 87% in fat and 41% in liver. The MRLs were subsequently derived by apportioning the ADI to the corrected total residues in fat and liver, in a ratio of 1.6:1. MRLs for cattle of 8 µg/kg in fat and 5 µg/kg in liver were derived in this way. The recommended MRL for cattle fat was rounded up to 10 µg/kg to reflect the uncertainty of the estimates of the bioactivity of the metabolites.

Maximum residue limits
In recommending MRLs for MGA, the Committee considered the following factors:

— The established ADI is 0–0.03 µg/kg bw, equivalent to 0–1.8 µg for a 60 kg person.
— The metabolites of MGA, according to tests in vitro using preparations from female cattle, were identified as 2β, 15β-dihydroxy-MGA (metabolite B), 6-hydroxymethyl-MGA (metabolite C), 15β-hydroxy-MGA (metabolite D), and 2β-hydroxy-MGA (metabolite E).
— Activation of steroid receptors by MGA and its metabolites in test systems in vitro was most selective for the human progesterone receptor, which is consistent with historical data in vivo.
— On the basis of the submitted data, the biological activity of MGA-related residues in edible tissues of beef heifers that have been fed with MGA is principally attributed to MGA.
— The most active metabolite of MGA, 2β-hydroxy-MGA (metabolite E), is nine times less potent than MGA.
— A suitable regulatory method is available.

On the basis of the above considerations, the Committee recommended MRLs in cattle of 8 µg/kg for fat and 5 µg/kg for liver, expressed as MGA.

These recommended MRLs would result in a theoretical daily maximum intake of residues as MGA equivalents of 1.8 µg per person, or 100% of the upper bound of the ADI.

Addenda to the toxicological monograph and residue evaluation were prepared.

3.8 Phoxim

Phoxim is an organophosphate insecticide used for topical treatment of cattle, sheep, goats and pigs. It was evaluated by JMPR in 1982 and

1984 (5, 6). At the fifty-second meeting of the Committee (Annex 1, reference 140), an ADI of 0–4 µg per kg bw was recommended for phoxim. The Committee recommended temporary MRLs of 50 µg/kg in muscle, liver and kidney tissues and 400 µg/kg in fat for cattle, pigs, sheep and goats.

On the basis of the new studies presented at the fifty-eighth meeting (Annex 1, reference 157), the Committee recommended permanent MRLs for edible tissues of sheep, pigs and goats of 50 µg/kg in muscle, 50 µg/kg in liver, 50 µg/kg in kidney, and 400 µg/kg in fat, expressed as phoxim. The Committee extended the temporary MRLs for edible tissues of cattle and requested submission of a residue depletion study for evaluation in 2004, to allow determination of the ratio of marker residue to total residue in cattle after topical application of the formulated product.

No new data were provided for evaluation by the Committee at its present meeting. The temporary MRLs for cattle were withdrawn.

3.9 Pirlimycin

Pirlimycin is a lincosamide antibiotic, closely related to lincomycin and clindamycin, that is active against Gram-positive bacteria, including *Staphylococcus aureus*, *Streptococcus agalactiae*, *Streptococcus dysgalactiae* and *Streptococcus uberis*, which cause mastitis in dairy cows. The general mechanism of action of the lincosamides is through binding to the 50S ribosomal subunit, thereby inhibiting peptidyl transferase, with subsequent inhibition of protein synthesis in susceptible bacteria. Pirlimycin is administered by daily intramammary infusion at a dose of 50 mg of free base equivalents per udder quarter, for 2 days. For extended therapy, daily treatment may be continued for up to 8 consecutive days. Pirlimycin has not been previously evaluated by the Committee.

Toxicological data
The Committee considered the results of studies on pharmacokinetics and metabolism, acute and short-term toxicity, genotoxicity, reproductive and developmental toxicity, microbiological effects, and studies in humans. Most of the studies of toxicity were carried out according to appropriate standards for study protocol and conduct. The studies of acute toxicity reported in the 1970s were conducted prior to the requirements for compliance with GLP and have no assurance of quality.

Pirlimycin, when administered orally as pirlimycin hydrochloride, appears to be poorly absorbed in rats. Approximately 5–6% of a radiolabelled dose was excreted in urine and >80% was recovered in faeces and gastrointestinal contents. Most of the radioactivity was present as pirlimycin and pirlimycin sulfoxide, the same compounds as those found in the livers of treated cows. Nucleotide adducts of pirlimycin and pirlimycin sulfoxide, formed by the activity of intestinal microflora, were detected in cows' faeces. These metabolites were not detected in rats but, because they are not found in edible tissues, they are not relevant for human risk assessment. Similarly, the bioavailability of pirlimycin in humans given an oral dose of pirlimycin hydrochloride appeared to be low.

The acute oral toxicity of pirlimycin hydrochloride was low. Signs of toxicity included depression, diarrhoea and gastrointestinal irritation. In rabbits, local application of pirlimycin hydrochloride resulted in severe ocular irritation and moderate dermal irritation at skin sites that had been abraded.

In a preliminary study, rats received pirlimycin hydrochloride at a dose of 0 or 500 mg/kg bw per day by gavage for 14 days. The treated group had lower liver weights and inflammatory changes in the gastric mucosa that were suggestive of irritation.

Rats were given pirlimycin hydrochloride at a dose of of 0, 50, 160 or 500 mg/kg bw per day by gavage for 30 days. Serum activities of aspartate amino trasferase (AST) and alanine transferase (ALT) were slightly higher in all treated groups but the increases were not proportional to the dose. At 500 mg/kg bw per day, a few myeloid bodies and an increase in lysosomes were found in hepatocytes. Inflammatory foci were present in the lining of the stomach in a few animals at 500 mg/kg bw per day and in one rat at 160 mg/kg bw per day. Since histopathology was not performed for animals treated with a dose of 50 mg/kg bw per day, a NOEL could not be identified.

Groups of rats were given pirlimycin hydrochloride at a dose of 0, 10, 30, 100 or 300 mg/kg bw per day by gavage for 91 days. In males receiving a dose of ≥30 mg/kg bw per day, there were decreases in serum total protein, albumin and globulin, and in liver weight. At 300 mg/kg bw per day, blood urea nitrogen was decreased in both sexes and kidney weights were lower in females. The NOEL was 10 mg/kg bw per day.

Two males and two females per dose were given pirlimycin hydrochloride in capsules at a daily dose of 0, 30, 100 or 300 mg/kg bw per day for 30 days. Both females in the group receiving 300 mg/kg bw per day showed frequent vomiting, excessive salivation and lost body weight, leading to the sacrifice of one female after 17 days. Serum activities of AST and ALT were elevated in the survivors at 300 mg/kg bw per day. Three dogs at 100 mg/kg bw per day and all dogs at 300 mg/kg bw per day exhibited liver changes consisting of centrilobular hydropic degeneration, and increases in lysosomes and myeloid bodies in the hepatocytes. The NOEL was 30 mg/kg bw per day.

Dogs were given pirlimycin hydrochloride in capsules at a dose of 0, 4, 16, 40 or 160 mg/kg bw per day for 92 days. Salivation and vomiting were increased at 40 and 160 mg/kg bw per day and serum activities of AST and ALT were elevated at 160 mg/kg bw per day. Inflammation and lymphoid hyperplasia of the stomach, which were suggestive of gastric irritation, were more severe in females given a dose of 40 and 160 mg/kg bw per day. The NOEL was 16 mg/kg bw per day.

Assays covering an appropriate range of genotoxic end-points were conducted *in vitro* and *in vivo* with pirlimycin hydrochloride. The results of all the assays were negative and the Committee concluded that the compound does not pose a genotoxic hazard.

Long-term studies were not carried out with pirlimycin and there are thus no data available on the carcinogenic potential of pirlimycin. However, the drug has no genotoxic potential, is not chemically related to known carcinogens and, in short-term studies, causes no changes that are likely to progress to neoplasia. The Committee therefore concluded that the drug is unlikely to pose a carcinogenic risk, and that studies of carcinogenicity were not necessary.

In a two-generation study of reproductive toxicity in rats, pirlimycin hydrochloride was administered at a dose of 0, 100, 200 or 400 mg/kg bw per day by gavage. Clinical signs of toxicity in adult animals included salivation, nasal discharge and urogenital/anogenital staining at doses of 200 and 400 mg/kg bw per day. The numbers of F_1 dams producing a litter were reduced at 200 and 400 mg/kg bw per day but the frequencies were at the lower end of the range for historical controls. Other fertility and reproduction parameters and the development of offspring were unaffected. The NOEL was 100 mg/kg bw per day.

Developmental toxicity was investigated in mice given pirlimycin hydrochloride at a dose of 0, 100, 400 or 1600 mg/kg bw per day by gavage on days 6–15 of gestation. Diarrhoea and soft stools were noted in dams at 1600 mg/kg bw per day. At this dose, fetal body weight was lower but development was unaffected. Pirlimycin was not teratogenic in mice. The NOEL for maternal and fetal toxicity was 400 mg/kg bw per day.

In a study of developmental toxicity in rats, pirlimycin hydrochloride was given at a dose of 0, 200, 400 or 800 mg/kg bw per day by gavage on days 6–15 of gestation. Soft stools, salivation and urogenital staining were observed at 400 and 800 mg/kg bw per day and body-weight gain was lower at 800 mg/kg bw per day. Fetal development was not affected at any dose. Pirlimycin was not teratogenic in rats. The NOEL for maternal toxicity was 200 mg/kg bw per day.

The most appropriate study to use in determining a toxicological NOEL was the 91-day study in rats. Hence, the NOEL for pirlimycin was 10 mg/kg bw per day on the basis of serum biochemical changes. As there were no long-term studies in animals on the toxicological effects of pirlimycin after prolonged exposure in the diet, an extra safety factor in addition to the usual safety factor of 100 was considered necessary. The Committee used a safety factor of 10 to account for the absence of a long-term study, leading to an overall safety factor of 1000. An ADI of 0–10 µg/kg bw was established on the basis of toxicological data.

Microbiological data
Pirlimycin hydrochloride has been tested for its inhibitory activity against microorganisms representative of the human colonic microflora. The most sensitive species were *Bifidobacterium* spp. and *Peptococcus/Peptostreptococcus* spp., with a minimum inhibitory concentration at which 50% of isolates are inhibited (MIC_{50}) of 0.12 µg/ml at an inoculum density of 10^{10} colony-forming units (CFU)/ml. In another experiment, strains of anaerobic bacteria at cell densities of 10^7–10^9 CFU were incubated with pirlimycin hydrochloride. Of the 36 strains tested, only three showed evidence of decreased viability at drug concentrations of 3 and 6 µg/ml. Pirlimycin sulfoxide and other unidentified metabolites showed lower or no activity against anaerobic bacteria.

In a model of pseudomembranous colitis in hamsters, single subcutaneous injections of pirlimycin hydrochloride were administered after oral treatment with *Clostridium difficile* as the colitis-producing agent. It was estimated that a dose of 2.6 mg/kg bw induced death in 50% of the treated animals.

Human volunteers received single oral doses of pirlimycin hydrochloride of 0, 50, 125, 250 and 500 mg, at weekly intervals. *Clostridium difficile* was found in the stool samples of two, four, five and three persons after each dose of the drug, and in one person in the control group. There were no effects on haematology, serum chemistry and urine analysis parameters.

A decision-tree for evaluating the potential effect of veterinary drug residues on human intestinal microflora was developed by the Committee at its fifty-second meeting (Annex 1, reference *140*). At its present meeting, the Committee used the decision-tree to answer the following questions in its assessment of pirlimycin:

Figure 1
Decision-tree for determining the potential adverse effects of residues of veterinary antimicrobial drugs on the human intestinal microflora

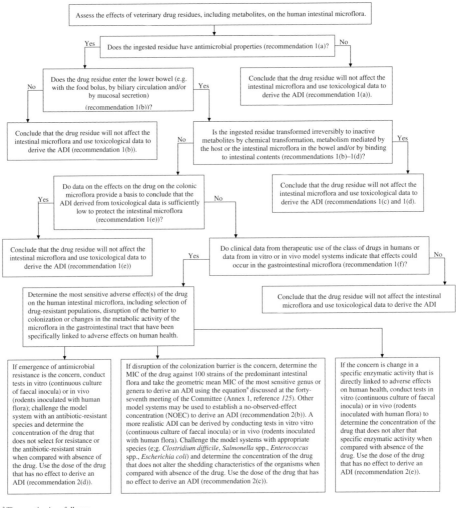

^{a} The equation is as follows:

Upper limit of ADI (µg/kg of bodyweight) = $\dfrac{\text{MIC (µg/g)} \times \text{Mass of colonic contents (g)}}{\text{Fraction of oral dose bioavailable} \times \text{Safety factor} \times \text{Weight of human (kg)}}$

where:

MIC_{50} = Minimum concentration of an antimicrobial drug completely inhibiting the growth of 50% of the cultures of a particular microorganism, as judged by the naked eye, after a given period of incubation. For the purpose of the evaluation, the MIC_{50} value is the mean MIC_{50} for the strain(s) of the relevant species tested. Alternatively, the lowest MIC_{50} value for the most sensitive species can be used.

Although MIC_{50} values are usually expressed in µg/ml, they are expressed as µg/g in this equation so that the ADI will be in µg/kg. When the MIC_{50} value is converted to these units, it is assumed that the density of the experimental medium is 1 g/ml.

A value of 220 g is used for the mass of the colonic contents and avalue of 60 kg is used for the weight of an adult. The safety factor used to take account of uncertainty about the amount and relevance of data available for review may range from 1 to 10. A value of 1 is used when extensive relevant microbiological data are provided.

1. *"Does the ingested residue have antimicrobial properties?"*
   Yes. Pirlimycin is a lincosamide that is active against Gram-positive aerobic and anaerobic cocci (eg. staphylococci, strepto-cocci, peptostreptococci) as well as Gram-negative anaerobes. Pirlimycin is the main residue in the milk of treated cows and pirlimycin sulfoxide is the main residue in the liver. The microbiological activity of pirlimycin sulfoxide is significantly less than that of pirlimycin.

2. *"Does the drug residue enter the lower bowel?"*
   Yes. Pirlimycin appears to be poorly absorbed in humans. Up to 34% of an oral dose was recovered in human faeces. However, since total recovery of the administered dose was only 40%, the fraction of the dose entering the colon is likely to be higher. A conservative estimate of the bioavailability of pirlimycin in the gastrointestinal tract would be 50%.

3. *"Is the ingested residue transformed irreversibly to inactive metabolites by chemical transformation, metabolism mediated by the host or intestinal microflora in the bowel and/or by binding to intestinal contents."*
   No. While there is no specific information on the nature of the substances excreted in human faeces, significant microbiological activity has been detected. Therefore, it is assumed that microbiological activity is likely to be present in the human gastrointestinal tract.

4. *"Do data on the effects of the drug on the colonic microflora provide a basis to conclude that the ADI derived from toxicological data is sufficiently low to protect the intestinal flora?"*
   No. A number of studies have demonstrated the potential for adverse effects of pirlimycin on the intestinal microflora. Studies of toxicity have not identified adverse findings at low oral doses and thus would not be expected to provide adequate protection for the intestinal flora.

5. *"Do clinical data from the therapeutic use of the class of drugs in humans or data from in vitro or in vivo model systems indicate that effects could occur in the gastrointestinal tract?"*
   Yes. Gastrointestinal effects (nausea, vomiting, abdominal cramps, diarrhoea) are the most commonly reported adverse reactions to the therapeutic use of lincosamides (clindamycin and lincomycin) in humans. Pirlimycin has not been used as a therapeutic agent in humans. However, limited experimentation in humans has revealed soft stools and overgrowth of *Clostridium difficile* in treated persons.

6. *"Determine the most sensitive adverse effect(s) of the drug on the human intestinal microflora."*

The available data indicate that oral exposure to pirlimycin is associated with disruption of the colonization barrier, rather than emergence of resistance. Other lincosamides are widely used in human medicine and also result in disruption of the colonization barrier. There are no studies available on the likely emergence of resistance to pirlimycin. In a study of the magnitude of and trends in the development of bacterial resistance to lincosamides, the pattern of susceptibility of human isolates of Gram-positive aerobic and anaerobic bacteria changed little over a 12-year period (1971–1983). It was concluded that disruption of the colonization barrier is the most appropriate end-point for the determination of a microbiological ADI.

7. *"If disruption of the colonization barrier is the concern, determine the MIC of the drug against 100 strains of predominant intestinal flora and take the geometric mean MIC of the most sensitive genus or genera to derive an ADI using the formula discussed at the forty-seventh meeting of the Committee (Annex 1, reference 125). Other model systems may be used to establish a no-observed-effect concentration to derive an ADI."*

Using all relevant data acquired in studies conducted in vitro and in vivo, the Committee considered that the study in humans was the most appropriate to use in determining a microbiological ADI. In this study, a single oral dose of 50 mg of pirlimycin caused a minor change in the intestinal microflora. A safety factor of 10 was used to address variability between human subjects. Because of the limited nature of the human studies (single oral doses, administration in males only, small sample size) the Committee considered that an additional safety factor of 10 was necessary, resulting in an overall safety factor of 100.

$$\text{Upper limit of ADI} = \frac{\text{NOEL}}{\text{SF} \times \text{BW}}$$

$$= \frac{50 \text{ mg}}{100 \times 60 \text{ kg bw}}$$

$$= 8.3 \,\mu\text{g/kg bw}$$

where:
BW = body weight
SF = safety factor

Evaluation
The Committee established a microbiological ADI of 0–8 μg/kg bw on

the basis of the NOEL for gastrointestinal effects in humans. The Committee rounded the value of the ADI to one significant figure, in accordance with current practice.

Data on pharmacokinetics and metabolism
Two studies in lactating cows examined the absorption, distribution, metabolism, and excretion of [^{14}C]pirlimycin after intramammary infusion. A third study was conducted to evaluate the bioavailability of [^{14}C]pirlimycin after intramammary administration.

In the first study, 12 lactating cows received an intramammary infusion of 200 mg of [^{14}C]pirlimycin per quarter (four times the recommended dose) into all four quarters, twice with an interval of 24 h. Total residues were measured in the whole blood, excreta, tissues, and milk. Peak mean blood concentrations of [^{14}C]pirlimycin were detected 6–12 h (119 and 126 µg/kg, respectively) after the second of the two doses. Although concentrations in the blood were low, some of the drug was absorbed into the systemic circulation. Residues in urine and feces accounted for approximately 10% and 24% of the administered dose, respectively. Eighty per cent of the residue in urine and 45% of the residue in faeces was pirlimycin.

In this study, residues in milk accounted for >50% of the administered dose. The depletion of total residue from the milk was bi-phasic, with a rapid initial phase attributed to unabsorbed pirlimycin being eliminated from the udder during the first three or four milkings after treatment. Milk samples were analysed by both a HPLC–thermospray–mass spectrometry (HPLC–TSP–MS) method and by a microbiological method to evaluate metabolites of pirlimycin. The results from the two assays are comparable and indicate that pirlimycin comprised nearly 95% of the total residue in the milk.

Animals in the study were slaughtered on day 4, 6, 14, or 28 after the last treatment. Residues in tissues accounted for <5% of the administered dose. Residues in cattle liver also were examined using the HPLC–TSP–MS and microbiological methods. The HPLC–TSP–MS analysis indicated that the liver residue consisted of two components only: pirlimycin sulfoxide as the major residue (76.5%) and unchanged pirlimycin as the minor residue (21.9%). The data demonstrate that the relative amounts varied over time, but were consistent at 4–6 days after the last treatment.

In the second study, 23 cows were treated with 50 mg of [^{14}C]pirlimycin per quarter udder into all four quarters, twice with an interval of 24 h. Cows were slaughtered on day 6, 10, 14, or 18 after the last dose. The disposition of the total administered dose in milk

(50.7%), urine (12.7%), faeces (27.6%) and tissues (4.6%) gave a recovery of 95.7% for the 18-day period. In this study, three components were found in the liver metabolite profile. These were identified as pirlimycin (24.5%), pirlimycin sulfoxide (61.8%), and pirlimycin sulfone (9.8%). In kidney, the mean composition of metabolites was 43.0% pirlimycin, 46.1% pirlimycin sulfoxide, and 7.2% pirlimycin sulfone. The composition of metabolites in the kidney is thus qualitatively similar to that in the liver.

In the third study, three lactating cows were treated intravenously with a single dose of 811 mg of [^{14}C]pirlimycin hydrochloride in sterile water. Blood samples were collected over a 7-day period. After an interval of 4 weeks, the same cows received an intramammary infusion of 790–795 mg of [^{14}C]pirlimycin, approximately 200 mg in each quarter. Blood samples were again collected during 7 days. In each study, milk, urine, and faeces were also collected for 7 days after treatment. All samples were assayed for total radioactivity and for pirlimycin. The bioavailability of pirlimycin in cattle after intramammary infusion in this study was calculated to be 34–41%.

The metabolites of pirlimycin in milk, tissues, urine and faeces have <1% of the microbiological activity of pirlimycin. Thus pirlimycin is the relevant residue from a microbiological perspective and is an appropriate marker analyte for residue monitoring purposes. On the basis of studies using radiolabelled drug, liver is the tissue with the highest total residues of pirlimycin and is a suitable target tissue for monitoring purposes.

Residue data
A residue depletion study was conducted to determine the concentrations of total residues and pirlimycin residues in the tissues of lactating cows after treatment with 50 mg of [^{14}C]pirlimycin per quarter into all four quarters, twice at an interval of 24 h. Cows were slaughtered and tissues were collected on days 6, 10, 14, and 18 after the last dose. Total residues were highest in liver, depleting from 2180 µg/kg in samples collected 6 days after the final dose to 890 µg/kg in samples collected 18 days after the final dose. Residues in kidney declined from 300 µg/kg at day 6 to 40 µg/kg at day 18. The concentration of total residue in the kidney was less than one-tenth that in the liver at 10 days or more after last treatment. Muscle and fat contained negligible concentrations of residue at all sampling times.

Four studies were conducted to evaluate the depletion of unlabelled pirlimycin in the tissues of cows treated under different regimes. There was an increase in pirlimycin residues in liver tissue during sample preparation in the first study. Therefore, the method was modified for subsequent studies to include a 24-h incubation step in liver tissue, which reduces pirlimycin sulfoxide to pirlimycin before sample extraction. The method was used to provide data to recommend a MRL for kidney and, as modified, a MRL for liver.

In the pivotal residue depletion study, four healthy cows were slaughtered at day 2, 7, 14, 21, or 28 after two treatments with 50 mg pirlimycin per quarter into all four quarters. Residues were determined for liver, kidney, muscle, and fat. As in other studies, residues were highest in liver, 1690 μg/kg, 2 days after last treatment, declining to below the LOQ of the method (25 μg/kg) 28 days after last treatment. Kidney residues were approximately 10–25% of the liver residues and were below the LOQ of the method (50 μg/kg) 14 days after last treatment. Residues in muscle and fat were below the LOQ of the method (50 μg/kg) at all sampling times.

All four studies provided data to evaluate depletion of unlabelled pirlimycin in cows' milk. As in the tissue analyses, residues were determined using either a microbiological assay or the HPLC–TSP–MS method. In all four studies, milk residues decline rapidly following cessation of treatment and were below the LOQ for the method (50 μg/kg) by approximately 72 h after the final treatment, irrespective of dose or mastitis status.

Effect on starter cultures
Studies were conducted to evaluate the effect of pirlimycin on starter cultures for cheeses, buttermilk/sour cream and yogurt. The Committee concluded that milk containing pirlimycin residues at <130 μg/kg would not affect production processes associated with starter cultures.

Analytical methods
Screening methods are available for the detection of pirlimycin in milk. These could be used to protect starter cultures.

A microbiological method has been validated for the quantitation of pirlimycin in milk and liver. The LOQ for the method is 20 μg/kg for the milk and liver.

An HPLC–TSP–MS method has been validated for the quantitation and confirmation of pirlimycin in milk and tissues. Preparation of the sample to be assayed has been modified to include an incubation step wherein samples of liver are stored at 37 °C for 24 h before extraction, reducing the sulfoxide metabolite to pirlimycin. While this incubation step may lead to an overestimation of the amount of pirlimycin residues present in the liver samples at collection, it ensures reproducibility in the analytical method. The quantitative method has an LOQ of 25 µg/kg for liver and 50 µg/kg for kidney, muscle, fat and milk. The lowest concentration at which the identity of pirlimycin can be confirmed is 100 µg/kg.

The Committee noted that the thermospray interface is no longer readily available. However, the method could be modified to use a currently available mass spectrometry interface.

Maximum residue limits
In recommending MRLs for pirlimycin, the Committee considered the following factors:

— An ADI of 0–8 µg/kg bw was established by the Committee based on a microbiological end-point. This ADI is equivalent to up to 480 µg for a 60 kg person.
— Liver contains the highest concentration of total residues and is the target tissue for residue monitoring purposes. Pirlimycin is the principle microbiologically active residue in tissues and in milk. In milk, pirlimycin accounts for nearly 95% of the total residues. Although pirlimycin sulfoxide represents a higher percentage (57–77%) of the total residues in liver than pirlimycin (22–25%), the microbiological activity of the sulfoxide is approximately 1% of that of pirlimycin. Therefore pirlimycin is the marker residue in both tissue and milk.
— A validated HPLC–TSP–MS analytical method was used to measure residues of pirlimycin in milk and tissues in the studies submitted for the Committee's review and would be suitable for monitoring residues for regulatory purposes, except for the limitation noted above.
— Concentrations of pirlimycin of <130 µg/kg had no effect on bacterial starter cultures used in the production of fermented milk products.
— The MRLs recommended for liver and kidney were based on residue data from the unlabelled residue depletion study as determined with the HPLC–TSP–MS method. The MRLs recommended for muscle, fat, and milk were based on twice the LOQ for the analytical method.

The Committee recommended permanent MRLs for pirlimycin in cattle of 1000 µg/kg in liver, 400 µg/kg in kidney, 100 µg/kg in muscle and fat, and 100 µg/kg in milk, determined as pirlimycin.

These recommended MRLs would result in a theoretical maximum daily intake of 305 µg or 64% of the upper bound of the ADI, based on the model daily food intake of 300 g muscle, 100 g liver, 50 g each of kidney and fat, and 1.5 kg of milk.

A toxicological monograph and residue evaluation were prepared.

3.10 Ractopamine

Ractopamine hydrochloride, a β-adrenoceptor agonist, is a phenethanolamine salt approved for use as a feed additive. The formulated products, which contain four stereoisomers of the compound, are recommended for use in finishing pigs, at a dose of 5–20 mg/kg of feed to improve feed efficiency and to increase weight gain, or at 10–20 mg/kg of feed to improve carcass leanness. The recommended dose for finishing cattle is 10–30 mg/kg of feed to improve feed efficiency and to increase weight gain and carcass leanness.

Ractopamine was previously evaluated by the Committee at its fortieth meeting (Annex 1, reference *105*). At that time, the Committee concluded that residues of ractopamine appeared to have little toxic potential and the effects recorded were mainly those to be expected from a β-adrenoceptor agonist. It might, therefore, be appropriate to assess ractopamine on the basis of a NOEL for pharmacological effects. However, because such a NOEL could not be determined, the Committee was not able to establish an ADI at that time. Before reviewing the compound again, the Committee wished to see further evidence and arguments pertaining to the perceived gaps in data on genotoxicity, carcinogenicity, pharmacology, and data in humans.

The present Committee considered additional data on the toxicity of ractopamine, including the results of studies of long-term toxicity, genotoxicity and carcinogenicity. Results of unpublished and published studies on pharmacodynamic and pharmacokinetic properties of ractopamine and other β-adrenoceptor agonists in animals and humans were also considered. All the pivotal studies were carried out according to appropriate standards for protocol and conduct.

Ractopamine is well absorbed in a number of animal species and rapidly excreted, with urine as the major route of excretion. Biliary excretion of ractopamine varies with species, with the highest percentage of the administered dose found in the bile of rats. In laboratory animals, the plasma half-life ranged from about 4 to 7 h. Absorption of orally administered radiolabelled ractopamine was ≥80% of the administered dose, as estimated by recovery of radioactivity in the urine and faeces of rats, dogs, monkeys, pigs and cattle over a collection period of up to 10 days. Only a minor fraction of radioactivity in the urine represented parent ractopamine. More parent drug was detected in rat urine after parenteral administration of [^{14}C]ractopamine than after oral administration, suggesting significant first-pass metabolism in the intestine and liver after oral administration.

In addition to the three major monoglucuronide metabolites, designated as metabolites A, B, and C, a fourth metabolite, D, was identified as a glucuronic acid diconjugate of ractopamine in the urine, liver and kidney of rats, dogs, pigs and cattle. In metabolite D, the glucuronic acid is attached to both hydroxyphenyl rings. Two minor metabolites, designated E and F, also found in all species, were not identified. The chromatographic profiles of radioactive extracts of urine and liver from rats, dogs, pigs and cattle given [^{14}C]ractopamine were qualitatively, but not quantitatively, similar for the same four glucuronide metabolites of ractopamine. A monosulphate conjugate and a sulphate/glucuronic acid diconjugate were identified as the major metabolites in the bile of rats. While the metabolites generally represented a greater fraction of the concentrations of residues in laboratory animals, it is concluded that dogs and rats used in the studies of toxicity were exposed to the same metabolites as those found in the edible tissues of pigs and cattle.

The results of a study in six healthy male human volunteers receiving a single oral dose of 40 mg of ractopamine hydrochloride indicate a similar profile of pharmacokinetics and biotransformation in humans and animals. Orally administered ractopamine was extensively and rapidly absorbed and low systemic concentrations of parent drug were found. The urinary metabolites were monoglucuronide and monosulphate conjugates. The half-life in plasma was about 4 h.

The Committee conducted a review of the literature and submitted data on the pharmacokinetics of β-adrenoceptor agonists in humans and in laboratory species, including those studies relevant to oral administration. The data suggest, for most compounds and species, rapid and extensive absorption from the gastrointestinal tract, significant first-pass metabolism, wide distribution to the tissues, and predominantly urinary excretion. Most β-adrenoceptor agonists have low lipophilicity at physiological pH. The metabolism of any given β-adrenoceptor agonist is similar in all the species studied and the major differences are quantitative rather than qualitative. In general, β-adrenoceptor agonists with halogenated aromatic ring systems (e.g. clenbuterol) are metabolized by oxidative and conjugative pathways and have long half-lives in plasma. β-adrenoceptor agonists with hydroxylated aromatic rings (e.g. ractopamine) are metabolized solely by conjugation and have relatively short half-lives. The pharmacokinetic data suggest that halogenated phenethanolamine β-adrenoceptor agonist residues comprising greater amounts of parent substance have a higher oral bioavailability and relatively slower rate of elimination and thus a greater oral potency than residues of hydroxylated β-adrenoceptor agonists.

In a long-term study of toxicity and carcinogenicity, CD1 mice were given diets containing ractopamine at a concentration equal to 0, 25, 130, or 840 mg/kg bw per day for males and 0, 35, 175, or 1085 mg/kg bw per day for females for 21 months. A significantly increased rate of mortality at the highest dose was attributed to the more severe cardiomyopathy observed in groups receiving the two higher doses. Dose-related decreases in body weight, body-weight gain, and food efficiency relative to controls could be anticipated after exposure to a β-adrenoceptor agonist with thermogenic activity. There was a dose-dependent increase in the incidence of uterine leiomyomas in female mice at 0 (1 out of 60 mice), 35 (5 out of 60), 175 (8 out of 60), and 1085 (10 out of 60) mg/kg bw per day. Treatment-related non-neo-plastic proliferative lesions of the female genital tract smooth muscle were not strictly dose-dependent. The NOEL was 25 mg/kg bw per day in male mice on the basis of changes in body weight and food consumption. No NOEL could be identified for the formation of uterine leiomyomas in females. A benchmark dose (BMD) was estimated as an alternative approach to a NOEL in order to define the point at which the incidence of leiomyoma in treated animals was higher than that in controls. The BMD was calculated as 201 mg/kg bw per day on the basis of an excess incidence of leiomyoma of 5% higher than in controls, and a 95% lower confidence limit.

In a 2-year study of toxicity and carcinogenicity, groups of 60 male and 60 female Fischer 344 rats received diets containing ractopamine at a dose equal to about 0, 2, 60, 200, or 400 (in females only) mg/kg bw per day. Survival was significantly increased in both sexes at the highest doses. Dose-related decreases relative to control in body weight, body-weight gain, and food efficiency were consistent with increased thermogenesis after exposure to a β-adrenoceptor agonist. Treatment-related morphological changes included an increased incidence of slight to moderate cardiomyopathy in females at the highest dose and in males at the two higher doses. Dose-related hyperplasia of the costo-uterine smooth muscle was observed in females at 0 (0 out of 60 mice), 2 (0 out of 60), 60 (3 out of 60), 200 (17 out of 60), and 400 (25 out of 60) mg/kg bw per day. No significant trends for neoplasm incidences in males were recorded. The only tumour that occurred at an increased incidence in females was the costo-uterine leiomyoma at 200 (6 out of 60) and 400 (27 out of 60) mg/kg bw per day; these tumours were not observed in other treated groups. The NOEL was 60 mg/kg bw per day in female rats on the basis of formation of costo-uterine leiomyomas. The NOEL was 2 mg/kg bw per day in male rats on the basis of enhanced cardiomyopathy.

The Committee noted that the induction of benign leiomyomas in mice and rats appears to be a general feature of β-adrenoceptor agonists, as shown by the prevention of the development of these tumours by co-administration of the β-adrenoceptor blocker propranolol in studies with other β-adrenoceptor agonists. The Committee considered, therefore, that ractopamine is not a direct carcinogen and the induction of leiomyomas is a non-genotoxic event with a threshold and concluded that all treatment-related effects observed in the long-term studies of toxicity in mice and rats were attributable to the β-adrenergic activity of ractopamine.

A 1-year study of toxicity was conducted in rhesus monkeys given ractopamine at a dose of 0, 0.125, 0.5, or 4 mg/kg bw by gavage once daily. No significant toxicological effects were recorded. A significant increase in body weight occurred in the animals at the highest dose. Monkeys treated with ractopamine developed tachycardia, with no other changes in the electrocardiogram. The heart rate was significantly increased in the groups given the two highest doses compared with controls; the maximum increase occurred during the first 4 h after dosing, and no significant slowing of the resting and nocturnal heart rates was seen. The heart weight relative to body weight was decreased at the two highest doses. β-adrenoceptor binding assays were conducted using the nonselective radioligand [^{3}H]dihydroalprenolol in membrane preparations made from heart and lung tissue. The affinity and number of β-adrenoceptors in the heart were not affected by ractopamine treatment, whereas there was a statistically significant decrease (23.8%) in the density of β-adrenoceptors in the lung in the group given the highest dose. The NOEL in this study in rhesus monkeys was 0.125 mg/kg bw per day on the basis of tachycardia.

In another study in which rhesus monkeys were treated with ractopamine at a dose of 0.25, 0.5, or 4.0 mg/kg bw per day by gavage for 6 weeks, assays with the radioligand [^{3}H]dihydroalprenolol at termination also revealed statistically significant decreases of 27.8% and 32.1%, respectively, in the density of β-adrenoceptors in the lung at the intermediate and the highest dose. No treatment-related effects on the affinity of β-adrenoceptors for the radioligand used were observed at any dose tested. The NOEL was 0.25 mg/kg bw per day on the basis of the decreased density of β-adrenoceptors in the lung.

The Committee noted that the two studies in monkeys could have underestimated ractopamine-induced β-adrenoceptor desensitization as measured by radioligand binding in preparations of tissue membranes. The Committee concluded, however, that β-adrenoceptor desensitization would not be induced at a NOEL at which β-adrenergic activity was virtually absent. Therefore, the NOEL for ractopamine was considered to be 0.125 mg/kg bw per day in monkeys.

The Committee further noted that ractopamine-induced cardiostimulation in monkeys occurred in the absence of cutaneous erythema and in the absence of clinical signs or microscopic lesions indicative of cardiotoxicity, thus suggesting that the cardiovascular response in monkeys differs from that in dogs. Dogs appear to be more sensitive than monkeys to vasodilation, hypotension, and reflex cardiostimulation, although the vasodilatory effects of ractopamine after oral administration have not been directly assessed in monkeys.

Ractopamine has been tested in a wide range of assays for genotoxicity. The compound gave negative results in a battery of prokaryotic and eukaryotic assays in vitro and test systems in vivo. Positive results were reported with and without metabolic activation in cytogenetic assays with cultured human whole blood lymphocytes in vitro, but not in a cell line derived from Chinese hamster ovary. Positive results were also obtained in the L5178Y thymidine kinase assay in lymphoma cells of mice in vitro, although ractopamine had given negative results in this assay in a previous study evaluated by the Committee at its fortieth meeting. It was suggested that the weak genotoxic effects observed in the assay in lymphoma cells of mice were mediated by oxidative stress induced by auto-oxidation of ractopamine to ractopamine–catechol and its further oxidation to a quinone in vitro. Co-incubation of antioxidants blocked the mutagenic effect of ractopamine and that of the positive control, epinephrine. Ractopamine did not induce aberrations in chromosomes or micronuclei of bone marrow cells when administered to mice and rats in vivo. The Committee concluded that ractopamine was not intrinsically genotoxic in vitro or in vivo.

Recently published studies indicate that the RR-isomer (butopamine) is the stereoisomer with the most activity at the β-adrenoceptor. Butopamine was shown to be a non-selective ligand at the $β_1$- and $β_2$-adrenoceptors, but signal transduction is more efficiently coupled through the $β_2$-adrenoceptor than the $β_1$-adrenoceptor. Therefore, the RR-isomer of ractopamine is considered to be a full agonist at the $β_2$-adrenoceptor and a partial agonist at the β_1-adrenoceptor. These results are consistent with the pharmacological characterization of racemic ractopamine in isolated cardiac (atria) and smooth muscle (costo-uterine, vas deferens, trachea), which shows a maximal response at β_2- and a submaximal response at β_1-adrenoceptors when compared with the full β_1- and β_2-adrenoceptor agonist isoproterenol.

In a study of acute cardiovascular effects, anaesthetized dogs were given a 10-min infusion of ractopamine at 35 µg/kg bw. All animals developed tachycardia (65% increases in heart rate) and decreased peripheral vascular resistance (67% decrease) with a fall in mean arterial pressure (50% decrease) during the infusion. Cardiac output increased by 50% as a result of the increase in heart rate, in spite of a decrease in left ventricular stroke volume. The decrease in stroke volume was accompanied by changes in the aortic flow waveform, consistent with an increase in left ventricular contractility. Upon cessation of infusion, the cardiovascular parameters returned towards control levels, but remained changed during the 30 min observation period.

In another study of acute cardiovascular toxicity, conscious dogs were given ractopamine as a single oral dose of 0, 2, 50, or 125 µg/kg bw. At the two higher doses, ractopamine caused dose-dependent increases in heart rate and left ventricular contractility, with maximum effects at about 2 h after dosing. There was a drop in both systolic and diastolic blood pressures during the 6 h period immediately after dosing. No significant changes were observed at the lowest dose. Dogs receiving the two highest doses demonstrated a slight abdominal skin erythema. The NOEL for this study was 2 µg/kg bw.

The acute cardiovascular effects of ractopamine were monitored in rhesus monkeys during a 10 min intravenous infusion of ractopamine at 35 µg/kg bw and a subsequent 30-min observation period. Heart rate increased about 20% during infusion and remained elevated throughout the monitoring period. Cardiac output, stroke volume and peak aortic flow increased by 35%, 14% and 80%, respectively, during the infusion and decreased steadily throughout the monitoring period. The aortic flow ejection period was shortened by 18% during the infusion and the monitoring period. Total peripheral resistance gradually decreased to approximately 70% of its initial value during the infusion and then slowly returned towards control values. In a second experiment in anaesthetized and conscious rhesus monkeys receiving this treatment, haemodynamic responses to ractopamine were not significantly affected by barbiturate anaesthesia.

The Committee noted that in studies of acute and short-term toxicity, dogs were more sensitive than monkeys to the cardiovascular effects of ractopamine. In both species, however, the relative contribution of direct stimulation of cardiac β_1- and β_2-adrenoceptors, and of reflex-mediated sympathetic effects reflecting the stimulation of peripheral β-adrenoceptors, to the overall cardiovascular effects of ractopamine is uncertain.

The dose-dependent effects of ractopamine on the human cardiovascular system were studied in a limited number of human volunteers (six persons) given ascending single oral doses equal to 67, 133, 200, 333, and 597 μg/kg bw, with an interval of 48 h between doses. Occasional mild to moderate sensations of increase in heart rate and heart pounding were reported at doses of 200, 333, and 597 μg/kg bw. Dose-dependent increases in heart rate and cardiac output, and shortened electromechanical systole, as measured by echocardiography, were observed. The changes appeared within the first hour after the administration of ractopamine and values gradually returned to those before treatment. The systolic blood pressure increased in a dose-dependent manner. Unlike in monkeys and dogs, ractopamine had little effect on diastolic blood pressure in humans. Only minor cardiovascular effects were observed at 133 μg/kg bw. The NOELs for the relevant cardiac variables were 67 μg/kg bw for electromechanical systole, ventricular ejection time, and maximum velocity of circumferential fibre shortening, 133 μg/kg bw for heart rate and 200 μg/kg bw for cardiac output.

The Committee concluded that the response in monkeys is more predictive of the acute cardiovascular response in humans exposed to dietary ractopamine than is that in dogs. Monitoring in the studies in animals and humans was appropriately timed to reveal the onset, time-to-peak, and duration of ractopamine-induced cardiac effects. The time course of the cardiostimulatory effects of ractopamine was comparable in humans, monkeys, and dogs.

The Committee reviewed publicly available literature on non-therapeutic effects in humans after long-term use of β-adrenoceptor agonists. The reported side-effects of prolonged therapeutic use of β-adrenoceptor agonists include tachycardia, vasodilation, skeletal muscle tremor, nervousness, metabolic disturbances (hyperglycaemia and hypokalaemia), and β-adrenoceptor desensitization. These effects are pharmacologically predictable, dose-related and potency-related, with cardiovascular effects being the most commonly reported side-effects. Non-pharmacological effects include airway hyper-responsiveness and increased airway inflammation. The incidence and severity of side-effects varies for any given compound. Tolerance to pharmacologically-predictable, non-therapeutic effects occurs readily. There is no evidence for any increased incidence of smooth muscle tumours such as leiomyomas, or of any other tumours, among human users of these drugs. Little or no relaxant response to β_2-adrenoceptor agonists has been reported for the non-pregnant human uterus. The potential side-effects of β-adrenoceptor agonists were adequately addressed in studies of the toxicity of ractopamine in laboratory animals and in humans, in order to predict the consequences of the intake of residues of ractopamine by consumers.

Evaluation

After reviewing the additional data on toxicology and pharmacology, the Committee reaffirmed the evaluation made by the Committee at its fortieth meeting, which stated that it was appropriate to assess ractopamine on the basis of a NOEL for pharmacological effects that are relevant to its ingestion by humans as a residue in meats.

The Committee concluded that the acute cardiac responses to ractopamine in humans were the most appropriate end-points for the calculation of an ADI. A combined NOEL of 67 μg/kg was determined on the basis of changes in electromechanical systole, left ventricular ejection time, and maximum velocity of circumferential fibre shortening. A safety factor of 10 was used to account for individual variability and an additional safety factor of 5 was considered appropriate to protect sensitive individuals and in view of the small sample size in the human volunteer study, thus resulting in a combined safety factor of 50. This approach provides a margin of safety of at least 20 000 times with respect to the formation of leiomyomas in mice and rats.

The Committee established an ADI for ractopamine of 0–1 μg/kg bw per day based on the NOEL of 67 μg/kg bw in the study in human volunteers and the application of a safety factor of 50, rounded to one significant figure.

Pharmacokinetic and metabolism data

Pigs. The Committee reviewed three studies in pigs. Two of these studies, which were reviewed previously by the Committee at its fortieth meeting, demonstrated that a steady state was achieved in 4 days on a diet containing [^{14}C]ractopamine hydrochloride and that pigs excreted 96.5% of the ractopamine-related radioactivity over the 7 days after the cessation of treatment. In a new study provided to the Committee at its present meeting, six pigs (each approximately 45 kg bw) were given feed containing [^{14}C]ractopamine hydrochloride at 30 mg/kg for 4 days and killed 12 h after the last dose. Free ractopamine accounted for 28.7% and 23.4% of the total extractable radioactivity in liver and kidney tissues. Metabolites A, B, C, D, E, and F represented 7.9, 10.4, 4.6, 5.0, 2.7, and 2.8%, respectively, of the remaining extractable radioactivity in the liver, and 11.0, 13.2, 22.3, 6.1, 1.4, and 1.9%, respectively, in the kidneys.

Cattle. The metabolism of ractopamine in cattle was investigated in a study in which a capsule containing [^{14}C]ractopamine hydrochloride at a dose equivalent to 45 mg/kg in feed was administered into the rumen. Metabolite C was the most abundant metabolite in cattle liver and kidney, while metabolite D, identified as glucuronic acid diconjugate of ractopamine, was the second most abundant metabolite in cattle liver and kidneys.

Residue data

Pigs. Five depletion studies in which pigs were given feed containing [^{14}C]ractopamine hydrochloride at various concentrations were considered by the Committee at its fortieth meeting. In two of these studies, total radioactive residues were compared with residues of free ractopamine. These studies demonstrated that the ratios of total residues to extractable non-conjugated ractopamine at 12, 24, 48 and 72 h were approximately 4:1, 7:1, 20:1 and 33:1 in livers, and 4:1, 4:1, 6:1 and 10:1 in kidney at the respective times after last treatment. Non-extractable residues accounted for approximately one-sixth of the total residues in both liver and kidney at 12 h. Total residues were 20 μg/kg or less in muscle and fat samples at 12 h after the last treatment with ractopamine, and were below the detection limits at subsequent time-points in all studies.

Five studies were reported that used unlabelled ractopamine hydro-chloride; three of these were considered by the Committee at its fortieth meeting. In a new study, pigs were given feed containing ractopamine hydrochloride at 15 mg/kg and were killed 12 h after the last feeding. The residue concentrations of ractopamine at 12 h were: kidney, 45 μg/kg, liver, 26 μg/kg; muscle, 5 μg/kg; fat, 1 μg/kg. In another new study, 36 pigs received feed containing ractopamine hydrochloride at 20 mg/kg for 10 days, after which groups of six pigs were killed at 12, 24, 36, 48, 60 and 72 h after the last exposure to medicated feed. Concentrations of ractopamine residues were 22 μg/kg in kidneys and 15 μg/kg in livers at 12 h after the removal of the medicated feed, and declined to 2 μg/kg in livers and 3 μg/kg in kidneys at 72 h. In addition, a preliminary report on the analysis of eyes from pigs killed at 12 and 72 h after final exposure to medicated feed demonstrated the presence of ractopamine residues, primarily in the retina, choroid and sclera, at mean concentrations of about 200 μg/kg.

The mean concentrations of ractopamine free base in liver and kidney, 11 and 24 µg/kg, respectively, were calculated from the pooled data from all studies in which pigs were slaughtered 12 h after the final administration of feed containing ractopamine hydrochloride at 20 mg/kg.

Cattle. Four studies of residue depletion in cattle were considered by the Committee at its present meeting. Six steers that received an oral dose of [^{14}C]ractopamine hydrochloride at 1.25 mg/kg bw twice daily for 7 days were slaughtered in pairs at 12 h, 4 or 7 days after final treatment. Analysis of liver, kidney, muscle and fat for total radioactivity revealed highest concentrations of residues at 12 h, as follows: liver, 1270 µg/kg; kidney, 970 µg/kg; muscle, 40 µg/kg; fat, 50 µg/kg. Total residues declined to 170 µg/kg in liver and 190 µg/kg in kidney on day 4, and 90 µg/kg in liver and 110 µg/kg in kidney on day 7. Muscle contained residues at 20 µg/kg on day 4, but no residues were detected in the remaining samples (the detection limit was approximately 20 µg/kg in all tissues). In a subsequent study, six steers and six heifers each received a gelatin capsule, administered into the rumen, containing [^{14}C]ractopamine hydrochloride at 1.12 mg/kg bw per day (a dose equivalent to 45 mg/kg in feed) for 7 days. Three animals were slaughtered at 12 h, or 2, 4 or 7 days after the last treatment. Total residues were determined in liver, kidney, muscle and fat from each animal. Residues of ractopamine were determined by liquid chromatography. At 12 h after final treatment, total residues in muscle and fat were approximately 20 and 10 µg/kg, respectively; no unmetabolized ractopamine was detectable. No residues were detected in muscle and fat from the subsequent sampling days. In liver at 12 h, concentrations of total and parent compound residues were 620 and 140 µg/kg, respectively, for a ratio of approximately 4:1. The equivalent results for kidney were 460 and 60 µg/kg, or a ratio of approximately 8:1. The ratio of total residues:parent residues in cattle tissues increased with time after final exposure to medicated feed.

In another study, three cattle received a gelatin capsule containing [^{14}C]ractopamine hydrochloride by insertion into the rumen, daily for 7 days. The dose was equivalent to consumption of feed containing 30 mg/kg of the drug. The animals were killed approximately 12 h after the final treatment and livers and kidneys were collected for analysis. The concentration of total residues found in liver was 250 µg/kg, 40 µg/kg of which was parent compound, while the concentration total residues in kidneys was 190 µg/kg, 40 µg/kg of which was parent compound. The ratio of total residue:marker residue at 12 h was approximately 6:1 for liver and 5:1 for kidney; this was similar to the findings in the previous study and in pigs. On the basis of these studies, the conversion factor for parent residue:total residues in beef liver at 12 h after last administration was 5:1, while in kidney a ratio of 6:1 was considered to be appropriate.

A study was reported in which a group of six cattle (three heifers, three steers) received feed containing ractopamine hydrochloride, in combination with monesin and tylosin, at 30 mg/kg for 14.5 days. The mean residue concentration of ractopamine in liver was 7 μg/kg at slaughter, 12 h after the last feeding. A group of six heifers received the same treatment regimen, with the addition of melengesterol acetate in the feed to give a dose of 0.5 mg per heifer per day. The mean concentration of ractopamine in the liver tissue from the heifers was 4 μg/kg at slaughter, 12 h after the final feeding. The primary purpose of this study was to demonstrate that the combination of drugs did not interfere with results of residue depletion.

In another recent study, six cattle received feed containing unlabelled ractopamine hydrochloride at 20 mg/kg (equivalent to 0.43 mg/kg bw per day) for 8 days. They were killed in pairs at 0, 3 and 7 days after changing to a non-medicated diet. Residues in liver and kidney, determined using the proposed regulatory method, at day 0 were 9 and 98 μg/kg, respectively, 3 μg/kg in both liver and kidney from one animal at day 3, and not detectable in the remaining tissue samples. Further analysis of the samples after glucuronidase treatment to convert glucuronides to free ractopamine indicated that ractopamine residue in the liver was 28 μg/kg at day 0. This suggested that the free ractopamine measured using the liquid chromatography–fluorescence method represented approximately one-third of the total parent and metabolites present. Using LC–MS/MS analysis, ractopamine residues were also found in retinal tissues of the cattle, at concentrations ranging from 1 to 2 μg/kg.

The Committee considered that hydrolysis of the metabolites to free ractopamine in the gastrointestinal tract after ingestion of residues in food could not be discounted and, therefore, the total residues are of toxicological concern. Since the analytical method measures only free ractopamine, and not the metabolites, a correction factor is required to adjust from marker to total residues. The appropriate correction factors were derived from the residue data at 12 h, which represents a practical minimum period from last consumption of feed containing ractopamine hydrochloride to slaughter. The data established that correction factors were only required for liver and kidney. In cattle, the correction factors are 5 to derive total residues from marker residues in liver, and 6 for kidney. The correction factor is 4 for pig kidney and liver. The Committee considered that a correction factor was not required to adjust marker residue to total residue in muscle and fat of pigs and cattle.

Analytical methods
Several validated ELISA procedures suitable for screening purposes were reported for detection of ractopamine residues at concentrations of 1 µg/kg in urine.

Analytical methodology used in the initial residue depletion studies was liquid chromatography with electrochemical detection. This method was the basis for the proposed regulatory method using fluorescence detection. The four stereoisomers co-elute as a single chromatographic peak. The method, which does not include an incubation to convert the glucuronide metabolites to free ractopamine, was validated in a multi-laboratory trial for pig tissues and later extended to include higher residue concentrations and edible tissues from cattle. Limits of quantification for the various tissues were 3–5 µg/kg. The method is suitable for regulatory use.

The confirmatory method proposed for regulatory use, based on LC–MS analysis of the extracts prepared for the determinative procedure, was successfully tested on both fortified and incurred liver and muscle samples. LC–MS/MS methodology using a glucuronidase incubation step to release glucuronide metabolites has also been reported for the detection of ractopamine residues in tissues and urine.

Maximum residue limits
In recommending MRLs for ractopamine, the Committee took into account the following factors:

— An ADI of 0–1 µg per kg bw was established by the Committee. This ADI is equivalent to 0–60 µg for a 60 kg person.
— The parent compound, ractopamine, is the appropriate marker residue.
— The appropriate target tissue for a routine monitoring programme is kidney.
— Suitable analytical methods are available for analysis of ractopamine residues in edible tissues of pigs and cattle.
— Maximum residue limit calculations are based on tissue residues at 12 h after administration, because animals treated with ractopamine will usually be slaughtered within 12–24 h of consumption of medicated feed.
— Maximum residue limits for liver and kidney of pigs and cattle were based on the mean residue concentrations of free ractopamine plus three standard deviations. The mean was calcu-

lated from the pooled data for pigs in all studies at 12h after the last feeding at the maximum recommended dose, 20mg/kg. These values for pigs were higher than the values for free ractopamine residues observed in cattle liver and kidney at 12h after administration.
— Factors to convert free ractopamine to total residues are 5 for liver and 6 for kidney of pigs and cattle. The factors derived at 12h after the last feeding were based on the results obtained in cattle, which provide a more conservative estimate of exposure.
— The maximum residue limits for muscle and fat are based on twice the LOQ. A correction factor to convert marker to total residues was not required.

On the basis of the above considerations, the Committee recommended the following MRLs for edible tissues of pigs and cattle, expressed as ractopamine base: muscle, 10µg/kg; liver, 40µg/kg; kidney, 90µg/kg; fat, 10µg/kg.

These recommended MRLs would result in a theoretical daily maximum intake of 50µg, or 84% of the upper bound of the ADI, based on a daily food intake of 300g of muscle, 100g of liver, 50g each of kidney and fat.

A toxicological monograph and residue evaluation were prepared.

4. Comments on chloramphenicol found at low levels in animal products

Chloramphenicol is a broad-spectrum antibiotic with historical veterinary uses in all major food-producing animals and with current uses in humans and companion animals. Chloramphenicol was previously evaluated by the Committee at its twelfth, thirty-second and forty-second meetings (Annex 1, references *17, 80* and *110*). A number of other agencies have also reviewed chloramphenicol (e.g. International Agency for Research on Cancer (IARC), 1990; European Committee for Veterinary Medicinal Products; United States Food and Drug Administration, 1985). Concerns have been expressed about the genotoxicity of chloramphenicol and its metabolites, its embryo- and fetotoxicity, its carcinogenic potential in humans and the lack of a dose–response relationship for aplastic anaemia in humans. Deficiencies identified in the data on toxicity of chloramphenicol include information necessary for the assessment of carcinogenicity and effects on reproduction. An ADI has never been allocated and consequently a MRL has not been assigned. This has resulted in the restriction of the use of chloramphenicol in veterinary medicine to non-food use.

Toxicological data

No toxicological data on chloramphenicol was submitted to the Committee at its present meeting. The current evaluation was made on the basis of an extensive review of the scientific literature, particularly that published since the forty-second meeting, and with a focus on the toxicological data in humans.

Reports on uptake and metabolism in humans and animals showed that chloramphenicol is rapidly absorbed when administered orally and that it is extensively metabolized. A study with human bone marrow in vitro also showed evidence of metabolism in this tissue.

A number of studies with chloramphenicol and several metabolites of chloramphenicol have shown that they are cytotoxic to bone marrow in vitro.

In order to assess the genotoxicity of chloramphenicol, the Committee reassessed the results of tests reported at its thirty-second and forty-second meetings, and also considered new studies available in the published literature. Chloramphenicol was shown to cause DNA damage in a human fibroblast cell line and in primary cultures of rat hepatocytes, but not in human bone marrow cells in vitro. The results of tests for reverse mutation in bacteria were mostly negative. In mammalian cells in vitro, chloramphenicol consistently gave positive results in tests for chromosomal aberrations, but results of tests for gene mutations and for sister chromatid exchange were inconsistent. Overall, these results indicated that chloramphenicol was genotoxic in vitro.

In tests for genotoxicity in vivo, chloramphenicol caused chromosomal aberrations in the bone marrow of mice, but gave negative results in tests for micronucleus formation in bone marrow of mice and rats. It is not clear why contrasting results were obtained in these two assays, but the Committee considered that it was prudent to regard chloramphenicol as a mutagen in somatic cells in vivo.

In data on heritable mutation reviewed by the Committee at previous meetings, chloramphenicol gave negative results in tests for dominant lethal mutation in mice and in *Drosophila melanogaster*.

At its present meeting, the Committee reviewed studies on genotoxicity with chloramphenicol and its metabolites in human bone marrow cells or peripheral blood lymphocytes in vitro. Only nitrosochloramphenicol and dehydrochloramphenicol induced DNA strand breaks, while chloramphenicol and other metabolites were without effects. This confirmed the results of previous studies that showed that some of the metabolites of chloramphenicol are genotoxic.

No adequate studies were available to evaluate the carcinogenicity of chloramphenicol in experimental animals. Chloramphenicol has been classified as "probably carcinogenic in humans" by IARC (7).

A number of toxicological studies in rodents were conducted in an effort to develop a model for chloramphenicol-induced aplastic anaemia in humans. While bone marrow depression was confirmed in these studies, it did not progress to the characteristic aplastic anaemia of humans and was therefore not considered to be a suitable model for the disease in humans. The reversible bone marrow depression that is seen in animals and humans receiving chloramphenicol can be attributed to its cytotoxicity.

A number of reports on epidemiological studies on the oral and injectable use of chloramphenicol in humans were reviewed; they confirmed that chloramphenicol was toxic to the bone marrow. In many cases, the toxic effects could be reversed by reducing or discontinuing treatment with chloramphenicol. There are, however, cases of aplastic anaemia that appear to be unrelated to dose and that are associated with a high mortality rate. In humans, the aplastic anaemia that is attributable to treatment with chloramphenicol is often fatal and is an idiosyncratic reaction that may have an immunological component. There is also evidence that some of the survivors of aplastic anaemia induced by chloramphenicol subsequently develop leukaemia.

The ophthalmic use of chloramphenicol represents the lowest therapeutic dose of the compound. Epidemiological data relating to the ophthalmic use of chloramphenicol in humans suggest that this form of administration is unlikely to be associated with aplastic anaemia. While any occurrence of aplastic anaemia associated with this form of administration is extremely rare, it is not possible to quantify the absolute risk of the ophthalmic use of chloramphenicol in humans because of the low background occurrence of idiopathic aplastic anaemia.

No adequate studies were available to fully assess potential reproductive toxicity with chloramphenicol. However, chloramphenicol has been shown to be embryotoxic and fetotoxic in a number of laboratory animal species.

In a case–control study in humans, the authors concluded that oral treatment with chloramphenicol in the second and third months of pregnancy presents little, if any, teratogenic risk. However, it is difficult to determine if any effects might occur during the first month of pregnancy.

Evaluation

As there is evidence that chloramphenicol is a genotoxin in vivo, it would be prudent to assume that chloramphenicol could cause some effects, such as cancer, through a genotoxic mechanism for which there is no identifiable threshold dose.

Epidemiological studies in humans show that treatment with chloramphenicol is associated with the induction of aplastic anaemia, which may be fatal. It was not possible to establish any dose–response relationship or threshold dose for the induction of aplastic anaemia.

The Committee noted that aplastic anaemia induced by chloramphenicol is a rare idiosyncratic response in humans, which may have an immunological component. In common with many other idiosyncratic immune system-mediated adverse reactions, no animal model could be developed. As a consequence of these considerations, and because the mechanism of chloramphenicol-induced aplastic anaemia remains unknown, the Committee could not identify any studies in animals or epidemiological studies that would assist the further toxicological evaluation of chloramphenicol.

The Committee concluded that it was not appropriate to establish an ADI for chloramphenicol.

A toxicological monograph was prepared.

Residue data

Most countries in the world do not permit the use of chloramphenicol in food-producing animals, in order to protect the health of consumers. Despite such restrictions, chloramphenicol has been detected in food samples collected in national monitoring programmes during the past 2 years and these residues have caused safety concerns. Shrimps, prawns, food products from aquatic animals, honey, royal jelly, meat and offal, sausage casings, rabbit and poultry meat and milk powder were amongst the commodities in which the drug was detected.

Chloramphenicol — an environmental contaminant?

While in some cases the results of monitoring clearly indicate intentional uses of chloramphenicol, it has also been argued that very low levels of chloramphenicol, such as those found in poultry and in products from aquaculture, could result from environmental contamination. The possibility that chloramphenicol could persist in the environment, or even be formed by soil microorganisms was discussed by the Fourteenth Session of CCRVDF, held in 2003 (2).

Chloramphenicol was first described as an antibiotic produced by cultures of an actinomycete isolated from soil by Ehrlich et al. (1947) (8). The soil samples were collected from a mulched field near Caracas, Venezuela, and from a compost soil on the horticultural farm of the Illinois Agricultural Experiment Station at Urbana. In studies conducted in 1952 (9), the adsorption, stability, and rate of production of chloramphenicol in soil under different laboratory conditions were determined. When sterilized soil was inoculated with *Streptomyces venezuelae* and was incubated for long periods, the presence in soil of chloramphenicol formed by the microorganism after a lag phase of several weeks was demonstrated. The highest concentration observed was 1.12 mg/kg. However, when workers of the same group and in the same year analysed samples of normal soils collected from 91 cultivated and grassland sites from nine states of the USA and from 13 other countries, no chloramphenicol was identified in extracts from these soils. In this initial study (1952), the limit of detection of chloramphenicol was 0.3 mg/kg (turbidimetric assay using *Shigella sonnei*). In other experiments with an improved limit of detection of 0.05 mg/kg, and including the 91 samples of the previous study, these results were confirmed. Chloramphenicol was found and identified in soils only when organic material was added before sterilization and seeding with *Streptomyces venezuela*.

Whether antibiotics are produced in soil in detectable amounts by indigenous soil organisms has remained a scientific dispute for several decades. It was only recently demonstrated that an antibiotic could be synthesized in detectable amounts in soil. Using biosensor methods with very low limits of detection, *Streptomyces rimosus* was found to produce oxytetracycline in untreated soil. However, similar studies have not been carried out for chloramphenicol.

With this background information and on the basis of an extensive search of the current literature, the Committee at its present meeting examined the following two hypothetical scenarios to explain potential environmental contamination of foods of animal origin with chloramphenicol.

Scenario 1
Assuming that:

— Chloramphenicol is naturally produced in the soil.

- Farm animals (e.g. pigs, chickens) ingest certain amounts of soil in their daily intake of dry matter.
- This may result in an uptake of chloramphenicol and subsequently in residues of chloramphenicol in tissues and products of those animals that are not associated with uses of chloramphenicol as a veterinary drug.

The Committee conducted a number of simple model calculations to estimate hypothetical intakes of chloramphenicol as a function of soil intake of animals. On the basis of data in the literature, it was assumed that 2% of the dry matter intake of pigs and chickens was soil. The concentration of chloramphenicol in soil was set at one of the following values:

- ≤0.05 mg/kg, corresponding to the limit of detection of the methods used by the authors of the historical studies, who were unable to detect chloramphenicol above this limit when they analysed a large number of soil samples from different countries; or
- 1 mg/kg, roughly corresponding to the highest concentration of chloramphenicol produced by *S. venezuelae* in inoculated sterilized soil samples supplemented with organic matter; or
- 25 mg/kg, roughly corresponding to the highest concentrations of chloramphenicol produced under experimental conditions with soils enhanced with tryptone and under the most favourable conditions.

The following steps were performed in the calculations:

- Calculation of average daily live weight gain;
- Calculation of daily dry matter intake as function of body weight/ live weight gain;
- Calculation of soil intake as a fixed fraction of dry matter intake;
- Calculation of chloramphenicol intake using the above assumed chloramphenicol concentrations in soil;
- Estimation of the resulting tissue concentrations on the basis of the known pharmacokinetic behaviour of chloramphenicol.

The Committee concluded that concentrations of chloramphenicol in soil, as they were found under laboratory conditions in the presence of organic material, would suffice to explain occasional traces of chloramphenicol in tissues and products of free-ranging and/or scavenging livestock animals. With the LOD achieved in the 1950s, however, it was not possible to demonstrate the production of detectable amounts of chloramphenicol in soil. No further empirical data have been obtained since 1952. The possibility that chloramphenicol, produced naturally by soil microorganisms, could lead to the residues found in food-producing animals cannot be ruled out, but remains an unexplored hypothesis that is currently not supported by experimental data.

Scenario 2
Assuming that:

— Residues observed are caused by the exposure of some food-producing animals to chloramphenicol that persists in the environment. Such environmental sources result from historical uses as veterinary drug.
— Any persisting residues of chloramphenicol in farm environments are most likely to originate from excreta of treated animals, and a possible source of contamination could be farming systems in which manure is used as fertilizer, e.g. in integrated farming. Integrated farming of fish/shrimp and livestock combines aquaculture with production of pigs, ducks, chickens, and/or other livestock animals. Manure produced by livestock may be used as soil fertilizer. Additionally, it is possible that manure may be used as a nutrient in fish/shrimp ponds. The nutrients contained in manure are taken up by bacteria and micro-algae, which themselves feed filtrating organisms, mostly zooplankton. Some of these organisms are then consumed by fish or shrimp.

The Committee reviewed published literature in order to investigate the conditions of integrated farming as a potential cause of chloramphenicol residues in food of animal origin. Chloramphenicol was in use in farm animals as a veterinary drug before authorizations were withdrawn in many countries and regions. Before these restrictions, significant amounts of manure, probably containing intact chloramphenicol, had been used as fertilizers. Concentrations of chloramphenicol in fresh manure and certain patterns of its use in integrated farming of aquatic species could, in principle, also explain low concentrations of residue in certain farm animals, such as scavenging chickens, free-ranging pigs and in aquatic animals. However, when reviewing the available information on the half-life of chloramphenicol under different environmental conditions, no evidence was found to show that chloramphenicol could persist in the environment for periods longer than several months, except in dry dusts. Therefore, if there was any risk of food contamination resulting from historical use in the farm environment these problems should disappear within several months of cessation of the use of chloramphenicol. Similar considerations apply to the persistence of chloramphenicol in aquaculture after past uses of the drug as medicated feed that had been directly applied in ponds.

Analytical methods

In the past decade, several methods were developed for the screening, quantification and confirmation of chloramphenicol in foods.

Screening for chloramphenicol could be performed with validated enzyme-linked immunosorbent assay (ELISA) kits. The majority of ELISA kits had a limit of detection of <1 μg/kg. However, confirmatory methods need to be used in order to avoid false positive results. For confirmatory purposes, highly sensitive methods based on GC–MS, either electron impact or negative chemical ionization mode, have been used. More recently, LC–MS/MS methods allow the determination and identification of chloramphenicol in food commodities such as honey, meat (chicken, turkey, pork and beef), fish and shellfish, at concentrations of <1 μg/kg. The limits of detection and of quantification are as low as 0.05 μg/kg and 0.1 μg/kg, respectively.

Conclusions

The Committee concluded that:

— There was no evidence supporting the hypothesis that chloramphenicol is synthesized naturally in detectable amounts in soil. Although this possibility is highly unlikely, data generated with modern analytical methods would be required to confirm this;

— There was evidence that the low concentrations of chloramphenicol detected by food monitoring programmes in the year 2002 could not originate from residues of chloramphenicol persisting in the environment after historical veterinary uses of the drug in food-producing animals. Owing to the high variability in the half-life of chloramphenicol under different environmental conditions, however, such a mechanism might occasionally cause low-level contamination in food.

Valid analytical methods are available to monitor low concentrations of chloramphenicol in foods; however, confirmatory methods require sophisticated and expensive equipment.

5. Future work

— The Committee suggested that a small working group, including experts from other JECFA and JMPR panels, should elaborate a set of phrases to be used to describe the Committee's conclusions on genotoxic and carcinogenic potentials, for discussion at the next meetings, and taking into consideration existing efforts. The working group should also address standard reporting for other toxicological end-points.

— The Committee encouraged the Secretariat to continue the development of a statistical tool for use when deriving MRLs for veterinary drugs whenever a suitable database is available.

— The Committee acknowledged that work is on-going within several Codex Committees on the terminology for analytical methods, and that this work is relevant for its own considerations. The Committee recommended that an expert be assigned to review on-going activites and to report at the next meeting.

6. Recommendations

1. Recognizing the potential public health consequences identified in this report (see 2.2.), the Committee requested early consideration by the Codex Committee on Residues of Veterinary Drugs (CCRVDF), in its role as risk manager, on how JECFA should proceed in the future in cases in which MRLs of lipid-soluble residues originating from the use of veterinary drugs are identified in milk. It should be noted that if CCRVDF indicated to the Committee that it should proceed in the manner described under chapter 2.2., it would be necessary for the Committee to reconsider its recommendations for MRLs for lipid-soluble residues in whole milk.

2. Recommendations relating to specific veterinary drugs, including ADIs and proposed MRLs, are given in section 3 and Annex 2.

3. The Committee at this meeting established a group ADI for cypermethrin and α-cypermethrin, and recommended that JMPR should consider if this approach is also relevant when such compounds are used as plant protection products.

4. For the MRL for pirlimycin, the Committee noted that the analytical method submitted by the sponsor had been validated suitably; however, the mass spectrometer interface was no longer commercially available and therefore the method would not comply with all Codex requirements for a regulatory analytical method. Since the Committee received information that verification of this method using different equipment was in progress, it recommended that CCRVDF should only propose the MRL for adoption by the Codex Alimentarius Commission if this work has been completed and made available to the Working Group on Methods of Analysis and Sampling in the CCRVDF.

Acknowledgement

The Committee wishes to thank Dr H. Mattock, St Jean d'Ardières, France, for her assistance in the preparation of the report.

References

1. *Residues of veterinary drugs in foods.* Report of a Joint FAO/WHO Expert Consultation. Rome, Food and Agriculture Organization of the United Nations, 1985 (FAO Food and Nutrition Paper, No. 32).

2. Codex Alimentarius Commission. *Report of the Fourteenth Session of the Codex Committee on Residues of Veterinary Drugs in Foods, Arlington VA, USA. 4–7 March 2003.* Rome, Food and Agriculture Organization of the United Nations (unpublished document ALINORM 03/31A).

3. *Pesticide residues in food — 1979. Report of the Joint Meeting of the FAO Panel of Experts on Pesticide Residues in Food and the Environment and the WHO Expert Group on Pesticide Residues.* Rome, Food and Agriculture Organization of the United Nations, 1980 (FAO Plant Production and Protection Paper, No. 26).

4. *Pesticide residues in food — 1981. Report of the Joint Meeting of the FAO Panel of Experts on Pesticide Residues in Food and the Environment and the WHO Expert Group on Pesticide Residues.* Rome, Food and Agriculture Organization of the United Nations, 1982 (FAO Plant Production and Protection Paper, No. 37).

5. *Pesticide residues in food — 1982. Report of the Joint Meeting of the FAO Panel of Experts on Pesticide Residues in Food and the Environment and the WHO Expert Group on Pesticide Residues.* Rome, Food and Agriculture Organization of the United Nations, 1982 (FAO Plant Production and Protection Paper, No. 46).

6. *Pesticide residues in food — 1984. Report of the Joint Meeting of the FAO Panel of Experts on Pesticide Residues in Food and the Environment and the WHO Expert Group on Pesticide Residues.* Rome, Food and Agriculture Organization of the United Nations, 1985 (FAO Plant Production and Protection Paper, No. 62).

7. *Monographs on the evaluation of carcinogenic risk of chemicals to man. Some pharmaceutical drugs.* Lyon, International Agency for Research on Cancer, 1990 (Vol. 50).

8. Ehrlich J, Bartz QR, Smith RM, Joslyn DA & Burkholder PR. (1947) Chloromycetin, a new antibiotic from a soil actinomycete. *Science*, 1947, **106**:417.

9. Ehrlich J, Anderson LE, Coffey GL & Gottlieb D. (1952) *Streptomyces venezuelae*: soil studies. *Antibiotics & Chemotherapy*, 1952, **2**:595–596.

Reports and other documents resulting from previous meetings of the Joint FAO/WHO Expert Committee on Food Additives

1. *General principles governing the use of food additives* (First report of the Joint FAO/WHO Expert Committee on Food Additives). FAO Nutrition Meetings Report Series, No. 15, 1957; WHO Technical Report Series, No. 129, 1957 (out of print).

2. *Procedures for the testing of intentional food additives to establish their safety for use* (Second report of the Joint FAO/WHO Expert Committee on Food Additives). FAO Nutrition Meetings Report Series, No. 17, 1958; WHO Technical Report Series, No. 144, 1958 (out of print).

3. *Specifications for identity and purity of food additives (antimicrobial preservatives and antioxidants)* (Third report of the Joint FAO/WHO Expert Committee on Food Additives). These specifications were subsequently revised and published as *Specifications for identity and purity of food additives*, Vol. I. *Antimicrobial preservatives and antioxidants*, Rome, Food and Agriculture Organization of the United Nations, 1962 (out of print).

4. *Specifications for identity and purity of food additives (food colours)* (Fourth report of the Joint FAO/WHO Expert Committee on Food Additives). These specifications were subsequently revised and published as *Specifications for identity and purity of food additives*, Vol. II. *Food colours*, Rome, Food and Agriculture Organization of the United Nations, 1963 (out of print).

5. *Evaluation of the carcinogenic hazards of food additives* (Fifth report of the Joint FAO/WHO Expert Committee on Food Additives). FAO Nutrition Meetings Report Series, No. 29, 1961; WHO Technical Report Series, No. 220, 1961 (out of print).

6. *Evaluation of the toxicity of a number of antimicrobials and antioxidants* (Sixth report of the Joint FAO/WHO Expert Committee on Food Additives). FAO Nutrition Meetings Report Series, No. 31, 1962; WHO Technical Report Series, No. 228, 1962 (out of print).

7. *Specifications for the identity and purity of food additives and their toxicological evaluation: emulsifiers, stabilizers, bleaching and maturing agents* (Seventh report of the Joint FAO/WHO Expert Committee on Food Additives). FAO Nutrition Meetings Series, No. 35, 1964; WHO Technical Report Series, No. 281, 1964 (out of print).

8. *Specifications for the identity and purity of food additives and their toxicological evaluation: food colours and some antimicrobials and antioxidants* (Eighth report of the Joint FAO/WHO Expert Committee on Food Additives). FAO Nutrition Meetings Series, No. 38, 1965; WHO Technical Report Series, No. 309, 1965 (out of print).

9. *Specifications for identity and purity and toxicological evaluation of some antimicrobials and antioxidants.* FAO Nutrition Meetings Report Series, No. 38A, 1965; WHO/Food Add/24.65 (out of print).

10. *Specifications for identity and purity and toxicological evaluation of food colours.* FAO Nutrition Meetings Report Series, No. 38B, 1966; WHO/Food Add/66.25.

11. *Specifications for the identity and purity of food additives and their toxicological evaluation: some antimicrobials, antioxidants, emulsifiers, stabilizers, flour*

treatment agents, acids, and bases (Ninth report of the Joint FAO/WHO Expert Committee on Food Additives). FAO Nutrition Meetings Series, No. 40, 1966; WHO Technical Report Series, No. 339, 1966 (out of print).

12. *Toxicological evaluation of some antimicrobials, antioxidants, emulsifiers, stabilizers, flour treatment agents, acids, and bases.* FAO Nutrition Meetings Report Series, No. 40A, B, C; WHO/Food Add/67.29.

13. *Specifications for the identity and purity of food additives and their toxicological evaluation: some emulsifiers and stabilizers and certain other substances* (Tenth report of the Joint FAO/WHO Expert Committee on Food Additives). FAO Nutrition Meetings Series, No. 43, 1967; WHO Technical Report Series, No. 373, 1967.

14. *Specifications for the identity and purity of food additives and their toxicological evaluation: some flavouring substances and non nutritive sweetening agents* (Eleventh report of the Joint FAO/WHO Expert Committee on Food Additives). FAO Nutrition Meetings Series, No. 44, 1968; WHO Technical Report Series, No. 383, 1968.

15. *Toxicological evaluation of some flavouring substances and non nutritive sweetening agents.* FAO Nutrition Meetings Report Series, No. 44A, 1968; WHO/Food Add/68.33.

16. *Specifications and criteria for identity and purity of some flavouring substances and non-nutritive sweetening agents.* FAO Nutrition Meetings Report Series, No. 44B, 1969; WHO/Food Add/69.31.

17. *Specifications for the identity and purity of food additives and their toxicological evaluation: some antibiotics* (Twelfth report of the Joint FAO/WHO Expert Committee on Food Additives). FAO Nutrition Meetings Series, No. 45, 1969; WHO Technical Report Series, No. 430, 1969.

18. *Specifications for the identity and purity of some antibiotics.* FAO Nutrition Meetings Series, No. 45A, 1969; WHO/Food Add/69.34.

19. *Specifications for the identity and purity of food additives and their toxicological evaluation: some food colours, emulsifiers, stabilizers, anticaking agents, and certain other substances* (Thirteenth report of the Joint FAO/WHO Expert Committee on Food Additives). FAO Nutrition Meetings Series, No. 46, 1970; WHO Technical Report Series, No. 445, 1970.

20. *Toxicological evaluation of some food colours, emulsifiers, stabilizers, anticaking agents, and certain other substances.* FAO Nutrition Meetings Report Series, No. 46A, 1970; WHO/Food Add/70.36.

21. *Specifications for the identity and purity of some food colours, emulsifiers, stabilizers, anticaking agents, and certain other food additives.* FAO Nutrition Meetings Report Series, No. 46B, 1970; WHO/Food Add/70.37.

22. *Evaluation of food additives: specifications for the identity and purity of food additives and their toxicological evaluation: some extraction solvents and certain other substances; and a review of the technological efficacy of some antimicrobial agents.* (Fourteenth report of the Joint FAO/WHO Expert Committee on Food Additives). FAO Nutrition Meetings Series, No. 48, 1971; WHO Technical Report Series, No. 462, 1971.

23. *Toxicological evaluation of some extraction solvents and certain other substances.* FAO Nutrition Meetings Report Series, No. 48A, 1971; WHO/Food Add/70.39.

24. *Specifications for the identity and purity of some extraction solvents and certain other substances.* FAO Nutrition Meetings Report Series, No. 48B, 1971; WHO/Food Add/70.40.

25. *A review of the technological efficacy of some antimicrobial agents.* FAO Nutrition Meetings Report Series, No. 48C, 1971; WHO/Food Add/70.41.
26. *Evaluation of food additives: some enzymes, modified starches, and certain other substances: Toxicological evaluations and specifications and a review of the technological efficacy of some antioxidants* (Fifteenth report of the Joint FAO/WHO Expert Committee on Food Additives). FAO Nutrition Meetings Series, No. 50, 1972; WHO Technical Report Series, No. 488, 1972.
27. *Toxicological evaluation of some enzymes, modified starches, and certain other substances.* FAO Nutrition Meetings Report Series, No. 50A, 1972; WHO Food Additives Series, No. 1, 1972.
28. *Specifications for the identity and purity of some enzymes and certain other substances.* FAO Nutrition Meetings Report Series, No. 50B, 1972; WHO Food Additives Series, No. 2, 1972.
29. *A review of the technological efficacy of some antioxidants and synergists.* FAO Nutrition Meetings Report Series, No. 50C, 1972; WHO Food Additives Series, No. 3, 1972.
30. *Evaluation of certain food additives and the contaminants mercury, lead, and cadmium* (Sixteenth report of the Joint FAO/WHO Expert Committee on Food Additives). FAO Nutrition Meetings Series, No. 51, 1972; WHO Technical Report Series, No. 505, 1972, and corrigendum.
31. *Evaluation of mercury, lead, cadmium and the food additives amaranth, diethylpyrocarbamate, and octyl gallate.* FAO Nutrition Meetings Report Series, No. 51A, 1972; WHO Food Additives Series, No. 4, 1972.
32. *Toxicological evaluation of certain food additives with a review of general principles and of specifications* (Seventeenth report of the Joint FAO/WHO Expert Committee on Food Additives). FAO Nutrition Meetings Series, No. 53, 1974; WHO Technical Report Series, No. 539, 1974, and corrigendum (out of print).
33. *Toxicological evaluation of some food additives including anticaking agents, antimicrobials, antioxidants, emulsifiers, and thickening agents.* FAO Nutrition Meetings Report Series, No. 53A, 1974; WHO Food Additives Series, No. 5, 1974.
34. *Specifications for identity and purity of thickening agents, anticaking agents, antimicrobials, antioxidants and emulsifiers.* FAO Food and Nutrition Paper, No. 4, 1978.
35. *Evaluation of certain food additives* (Eighteenth report of the Joint FAO/WHO Expert Committee on Food Additives). FAO Nutrition Meetings Series, No. 54, 1974; WHO Technical Report Series, No. 557, 1974, and corrigendum.
36. *Toxicological evaluation of some food colours, enzymes, flavour enhancers, thickening agents, and certain other food additives.* FAO Nutrition Meetings Report Series, No. 54A, 1975; WHO Food Additives Series, No. 6, 1975.
37. *Specifications for the identity and purity of some food colours, enhancers, thickening agents, and certain food additives.* FAO Nutrition Meetings Report Series, No. 54B, 1975; WHO Food Additives Series, No. 7, 1975.
38. *Evaluation of certain food additives: some food colours, thickening agents, smoke condensates, and certain other substances.* (Nineteenth report of the Joint FAO/WHO Expert Committee on Food Additives). FAO Nutrition Meetings Series, No. 55, 1975; WHO Technical Report Series, No. 576, 1975.
39. *Toxicological evaluation of some food colours, thickening agents, and certain other substances.* FAO Nutrition Meetings Report Series, No. 55A, 1975; WHO Food Additives Series, No. 8, 1975.

40. *Specifications for the identity and purity of certain food additives.* FAO Nutrition Meetings Report Series, No. 55B, 1976; WHO Food Additives Series, No. 9, 1976.

41. *Evaluation of certain food additives* (Twentieth report of the Joint FAO/WHO Expert Committee on Food Additives). FAO Food and Nutrition Meetings Series, No. 1, 1976; WHO Technical Report Series, No. 599, 1976.

42. *Toxicological evaluation of certain food additives.* WHO Food Additives Series, No. 10, 1976.

43. *Specifications for the identity and purity of some food additives.* FAO Food and Nutrition Series, No. 1B, 1977; WHO Food Additives Series, No. 11, 1977.

44. *Evaluation of certain food additives* (Twenty-first report of the Joint FAO/WHO Expert Committee on Food Additives). WHO Technical Report Series, No. 617, 1978.

45. *Summary of toxicological data of certain food additives.* WHO Food Additives Series, No. 12, 1977.

46. *Specifications for identity and purity of some food additives, including antioxidant, food colours, thickeners, and others.* FAO Nutrition Meetings Report Series, No. 57, 1977.

47. *Evaluation of certain food additives and contaminants* (Twenty-second report of the Joint FAO/WHO Expert Committee on Food Additives). WHO Technical Report Series, No. 631, 1978.

48. *Summary of toxicological data of certain food additives and contaminants.* WHO Food Additives Series, No. 13, 1978.

49. *Specifications for the identity and purity of certain food additives.* FAO Food and Nutrition Paper, No. 7, 1978.

50. *Evaluation of certain food additives* (Twenty-third report of the Joint FAO/WHO Expert Committee on Food Additives). WHO Technical Report Series, No. 648, 1980, and corrigenda.

51. *Toxicological evaluation of certain food additives.* WHO Food Additives Series, No. 14, 1980.

52. *Specifications for identity and purity of food colours, flavouring agents, and other food additives.* FAO Food and Nutrition Paper, No. 12, 1979.

53. *Evaluation of certain food additives* (Twenty-fourth report of the Joint FAO/WHO Expert Committee on Food Additives). WHO Technical Report Series, No. 653, 1980.

54. *Toxicological evaluation of certain food additives.* WHO Food Additives Series, No. 15, 1980.

55. *Specifications for identity and purity of food additives (sweetening agents, emulsifying agents, and other food additives).* FAO Food and Nutrition Paper, No. 17, 1980.

56. *Evaluation of certain food additives* (Twenty-fifth report of the Joint FAO/WHO Expert Committee on Food Additives). WHO Technical Report Series, No. 669, 1981.

57. *Toxicological evaluation of certain food additives.* WHO Food Additives Series, No. 16, 1981.

58. *Specifications for identity and purity of food additives (carrier solvents, emulsifiers and stabilizers, enzyme preparations, flavouring agents, food colours, sweetening agents, and other food additives).* FAO Food and Nutrition Paper, No. 19, 1981.

59. *Evaluation of certain food additives and contaminants* (Twenty-sixth report of the Joint FAO/WHO Expert Committee on Food Additives). WHO Technical Report Series, No. 683, 1982.

60. *Toxicological evaluation of certain food additives.* WHO Food Additives Series, No. 17, 1982.
61. *Specifications for the identity and purity of certain food additives.* FAO Food and Nutrition Paper, No. 25, 1982.
62. *Evaluation of certain food additives and contaminants* (Twenty-seventh report of the Joint FAO/WHO Expert Committee on Food Additives). WHO Technical Report Series, No. 696, 1983, and corrigenda.
63. *Toxicological evaluation of certain food additives and contaminants.* WHO Food Additives Series, No. 18, 1983.
64. *Specifications for the identity and purity of certain food additives.* FAO Food and Nutrition Paper, No. 28, 1983.
65. *Guide to specifications General notices, general methods, identification tests, test solutions, and other reference materials.* FAO Food and Nutrition Paper, No. 5, Rev. 1, 1983.
66. *Evaluation of certain food additives and contaminants* (Twenty-eighth report of the Joint FAO/WHO Expert Committee on Food Additives). WHO Technical Report Series, No. 710, 1984, and corrigendum.
67. *Toxicological evaluation of certain food additives and contaminants.* WHO Food Additives Series, No. 19, 1984.
68. *Specifications for the identity and purity of food colours.* FAO Food and Nutrition Paper, No. 31/1, 1984.
69. *Specifications for the identity and purity of food additives.* FAO Food and Nutrition Paper, No. 31/2, 1984.
70. *Evaluation of certain food additives and contaminants* (Twenty-ninth report of the Joint FAO/WHO Expert Committee on Food Additives). WHO Technical Report Series, No. 733, 1986, and corrigendum.
71. *Specifications for the identity and purity of certain food additives.* FAO Food and Nutrition Paper, No. 34, 1986.
72. *Toxicological evaluation of certain food additives and contaminants.* WHO Food Additives Series, No. 20. Cambridge University Press, 1987.
73. *Evaluation of certain food additives and contaminants* (Thirtieth report of the Joint FAO/WHO Expert Committee on Food Additives). WHO Technical Report Series, No. 751, 1987.
74. *Toxicological evaluation of certain food additives and contaminants.* WHO Food Additives Series, No. 21. Cambridge University Press, 1987.
75. *Specifications for the identity and purity of certain food additives.* FAO Food and Nutrition Paper, No. 37, 1986.
76. *Principles for the safety assessment of food additives and contaminants in food.* WHO Environmental Health Criteria, No. 70. Geneva, World Health Organization, 1987 (out of print). The full text is available electronically at www.who.int/pcs.
77. *Evaluation of certain food additives and contaminants* (Thirty-first report of the Joint FAO/WHO Expert Committee on Food Additives). WHO Technical Report Series, No. 759, 1987 and corrigendum.
78. *Toxicological evaluation of certain food additives.* WHO Food Additives Series, No. 22. Cambridge University Press, 1988.
79. *Specifications for the identity and purity of certain food additives.* FAO Food and Nutrition Paper, No. 38, 1988.
80. *Evaluation of certain veterinary drug residues in food* (Thirty-second report of the Joint FAO/WHO Expert Committee on Food Additives). WHO Technical Report Series, No. 763, 1988.

81. *Toxicological evaluation of certain veterinary drug residues in food.* WHO Food Additives Series, No. 23. Cambridge University Press, 1988.

82. *Residues of some veterinary drugs in animals and foods.* FAO Food and Nutrition Paper, No. 41, 1988.

83. *Evaluation of certain food additives and contaminants* (Thirty-third report of the Joint FAO/WHO Expert Committee on Food Additives). WHO Technical Report Series, No. 776, 1989.

84. *Toxicological evaluation of certain food additives and contaminants.* WHO Food Additives Series, No. 24. Cambridge University Press, 1989.

85. *Evaluation of certain veterinary drug residues in food* (Thirty-fourth report of the Joint FAO/WHO Expert Committee on Food Additives). WHO Technical Report Series, No. 788, 1989.

86. *Toxicological evaluation of certain veterinary drug residues in food.* WHO Food Additives Series, No. 25, 1990.

87. *Residues of some veterinary drugs in animals and foods.* FAO Food and Nutrition Paper, No. 41/2, 1990.

88. *Evaluation of certain food additives and contaminants* (Thirty-fifth report of the Joint FAO/WHO Expert Committee on Food Additives). WHO Technical Report Series, No. 789, 1990, and corrigenda.

89. *Toxicological evaluation of certain food additives and contaminants.* WHO Food Additives Series, No. 26, 1990.

90. *Specifications for identity and purity of certain food additives.* FAO Food and Nutrition Paper, No. 49, 1990.

91. *Evaluation of certain veterinary drug residues in food* (Thirty-sixth report of the Joint FAO/WHO Expert Committee on Food Additives). WHO Technical Report Series, No. 799, 1990.

92. *Toxicological evaluation of certain veterinary drug residues in food.* WHO Food Additives Series, No. 27, 1991.

93. *Residues of some veterinary drugs in animals and foods.* FAO Food and Nutrition Paper, No. 41/3, 1991.

94. *Evaluation of certain food additives and contaminants* (Thirty-seventh report of the Joint FAO/WHO Expert Committee on Food Additives). WHO Technical Report Series, No. 806, 1991, and corrigenda.

95. *Toxicological evaluation of certain food additives and contaminants.* WHO Food Additives Series, No. 28, 1991.

96. *Compendium of food additive specifications (Joint FAO/WHO Expert Committee on Food Additives (JECFA)). Combined specifications from 1st through the 37th meetings, 1956–1990.* Rome, Food and Agricultural Organization of the United Nations, 1992 (2 volumes).

97. *Evaluation of certain veterinary drug residues in food* (Thirty-eighth report of the Joint FAO/WHO Expert Committee on Food Additives). WHO Technical Report Series, No. 815, 1991.

98. *Toxicological evaluation of certain veterinary residues in food.* WHO Food Additives Series, No. 29, 1991.

99. *Residues of some veterinary drugs in animals and foods.* FAO Food and Nutrition Paper, No. 41/4, 1991.

100. *Guide to specifications — General notices, general analytical techniques, identification tests, test solutions, and other reference materials.* FAO Food and Nutrition Paper, No. 5, Ref. 2, 1991.

101. *Evaluation of certain food additives and naturally occurring toxicants* (Thirty-ninth report of the Joint FAO/WHO Expert Committee on Food Additives). WHO Technical Report Series No. 828, 1992.

102. *Toxicological evaluation of certain food additives and naturally occurring toxicants.* WHO Food Additive Series, No. 30, 1993.
103. *Compendium of food additive specifications: addendum 1.* FAO Food and Nutrition Paper, No. 52, 1992.
104. *Evaluation of certain veterinary drug residues in food* (Fortieth report of the Joint FAO/WHO Expert Committee on Food Additives). WHO Technical Report Series, No. 832, 1993.
105. *Toxicological evaluation of certain veterinary drug residues in food.* WHO Food Additives Series, No. 31, 1993.
106. *Residues of some veterinary drugs in animals and food.* FAO Food and Nutrition Paper, No. 41/5, 1993.
107. *Evaluation of certain food additives and contaminants* (Forty-first report of the Joint FAO/WHO Expert Committee on Food Additives). WHO Technical Report Series, No. 837, 1993.
108. *Toxicological evaluation of certain food additives and contaminants.* WHO Food Additives Series, No. 32, 1993.
109. *Compendium of food additive specifications: addendum 2.* FAO Food and Nutrition Paper, No. 52, Add. 2, 1993.
110. *Evaluation of certain veterinary drug residues in food* (Forty-second report of the Joint FAO/WHO Expert Committee on Food Additives). WHO Technical Report Series, No. 851, 1995.
111. *Toxicological evaluation of certain veterinary drug residues in food.* WHO Food Additives Series, No. 33, 1994.
112. *Residues of some veterinary drugs in animals and foods.* FAO Food and Nutrition Paper, No. 41/6, 1994.
113. *Evaluation of certain veterinary drug residues in food* (Forty-third report of the Joint FAO/WHO Expert Committee on Food Additives). WHO Technical Report Series, No. 855, 1995, and corrigendum.
114. *Toxicological evaluation of certain veterinary drug residues in food.* WHO Food Additives Series, No. 34, 1995.
115. *Residues of some veterinary drugs in animals and foods.* FAO Food and Nutrition Paper, No. 41/7, 1995.
116. *Evaluation of certain food additives and contaminants* (Forty-fourth report of the Joint FAO/WHO Expert Committee on Food Additives). WHO Technical Report Series, No. 859, 1995.
117. *Toxicological evaluation of certain food additives and contaminants.* WHO Food Additives Series, No. 35, 1996.
118. *Compendium of food additive specifications: addendum 3.* FAO Food and Nutrition Paper, No. 52, Add. 3, 1995.
119. *Evaluation of certain veterinary drug residues in food* (Forty-fifth report of the Joint FAO/WHO Expert Committee on Food Additives). WHO Technical Report Series, No. 864, 1996.
120. *Toxicological evaluation of certain veterinary drug residues in food.* WHO Food Additives Series, No. 36, 1996.
121. *Residues of some veterinary drugs in animals and foods.* FAO Food and Nutrition Paper, No. 41/8, 1996.
122. *Evaluation of certain food additives and contaminants* (Forty-sixth report of the Joint FAO/WHO Expert Committee on Food Additives). WHO Technical Report Series, No. 868, 1997.
123. *Toxicological evaluation of certain food additives.* WHO Food Additives Series, No. 37, 1996.

124. *Compendium of food additive specifications, addendum 4.* FAO Food and Nutrition Paper, No. 52, Add. 4, 1996.

125. *Evaluation of certain veterinary drug residues in food* (Forty-seventh report of the Joint FAO/WHO Expert Committee on Food Additives). WHO Technical Report Series, No. 876, 1998.

126. *Toxicological evaluation of certain veterinary drug residues in food.* WHO Food Additives Series, No. 38, 1996.

127. *Residues of some veterinary drugs in animals and foods.* FAO Food and Nutrition Paper, No. 41/9, 1997.

128. *Evaluation of certain veterinary drug residues in food* (Forty-eighth report of the Joint FAO/WHO Expert Committee on Food Additives). WHO Technical Report Series, No. 879, 1998.

129. *Toxicological evaluation of certain veterinary drug residues in food.* WHO Food Additives Series, No. 39, 1997.

130. *Residues of some veterinary drugs in animals and foods.* FAO Food and Nutrition Paper, No. 41/10, 1998.

131. *Evaluation of certain food additives and contaminants* (Forty-ninth report of the Joint FAO/WHO Expert Committee on Food Additives). WHO Technical Report Series, No. 884, 1999.

132. *Safety evaluation of certain food additives and contaminants.* WHO Food Additives Series, No. 40, 1998.

133. *Compendium of food additive specifications: addendum 5.* FAO Food and Nutrition Paper, No. 52, Add. 5, 1997.

134. *Evaluation of certain veterinary drug residues in food* (Fiftieth report of the Joint FAO/WHO Expert Committee on Food Additives). WHO Technical Report Series, No. 888, 1999.

135. *Toxicological evaluation of certain veterinary drug residues in food.* WHO Food Additives Series, No. 41, 1998.

136. *Residues of some veterinary drugs in animals and foods.* FAO Food and Nutrition Paper, No. 41/11, 1999.

137. *Evaluation of certain food additives* (Fifty-first report of the Joint FAO/WHO Expert Committee on Food Additives). WHO Technical Report Series, No. 891, 2000.

138. *Safety evaluation of certain food additives.* WHO Food Additives Series, No. 42, 1999.

139. *Compendium of food additive specifications, addendum 6.* FAO Food and Nutrition Paper, No. 52, Add. 6, 1998.

140. *Evaluation of certain veterinary drug residues in food* (Fifty-second report of the Joint FAO/WHO Expert Committee on Food Additives). WHO Technical Report Series, No. 893, 2000.

141. *Toxicological evaluation of certain veterinary drug residues in food.* WHO Food Additives Series, No. 43, 2000

142. *Residues of some veterinary drugs in animals and foods.* FAO Food and Nutrition Paper, No. 41/12, 2000.

143. *Evaluation of certain food additives and contaminants* (Fifty-third report of the Joint FAO/WHO Expert Committee on Food Additives). WHO Technical Report Series, No. 896, 2000

144. *Safety evaluation of certain food additives and contaminants.* WHO Food Additives Series, No. 44, 2000.

145. *Compendium of food additive specifications, addendum 7.* FAO Food and Nutrition Paper, No. 52, Add. 7, 1999.

146. *Evaluation of certain veterinary drug residues in food* (Fifty-fourth report of the Joint FAO/WHO Expert Committee on Food Additives). WHO Technical Report Series, No. 900, 2001

147. *Toxicological evaluation of certain veterinary drug residues in food.* WHO Food Additives Series, No. 45, 2000.

148. *Residues of some veterinary drugs in animals and foods.* FAO Food and Nutrition Paper, No. 41/13, 2000.

149. *Evaluation of certain food additives and contaminants* (Fifty-fifth report of the Joint FAO/WHO Expert Committee on Food Additives). WHO Technical Report Series No. 901, 2001.

150. *Safety evaluation of certain food additives and contaminants.* WHO Food Additives Series, No. 46, 2001.

151. *Compendium of food additive specifications: addendum 8.* FAO Food and Nutrition Paper, No. 52, Add. 8, 2000.

152. *Evaluation of certain mycotoxins in food* (Fifty-sixth report of the Joint FAO/WHO Expert Committee on Food Additives). WHO Technical Report Series No. 906, 2002.

153. *Safety evaluation of certain mycotoxins in food.* WHO Food Additives Series, No. 47/FAO Food and Nutrition Paper 74, 2001.

154. *Evaluation of certain food additives and contaminants* (Fifty-seventh report of the Joint FAO/WHO Expert Committee on Food Additives). WHO Technical Report Series, No. 909, 2002.

155. *Safety evaluation of certain food additives and contaminants.* WHO Food Additives Series, No. 48, 2002.

156. *Compendium of food additive specifications: addendum 9.* FAO Food and Nutrition Paper, No. 52, Add. 9, 2001.

157. *Evaluation of certain veterinary drug residues in food* (Fifty-eighth report of the Joint FAO/WHO Expert Committee on Food Additives). WHO Technical Report Series, No. 911, 2002.

158. *Toxicological evaluation of certain veterinary drug residues in food.* WHO Food Additives Series, No. 49, 2002.

159. *Residues of some veterinary drugs in animals and foods.* FAO Food and Nutrition Paper, No. 41/14, 2002.

160. *Evaluation of certain food additives and contaminants* (Fifty-ninth report of the Joint FAO/WHO Expert Committee on Food Additives). WHO Technical Report Series, No. 913, 2002.

162. *Safety evaluation of certain food additives and contaminants.* WHO Food Additives Series, No. 50, 2003.

163. *Evaluation of certain veterinary drug residues in food* (Sixtieth report of the Joint FAO/WHO Expert Committee on Food Additives). WHO Technical Report Series, No. 918, 2003.

164. *Toxicological evaluation of certain veterinary drug residues in food.* WHO Food Additives Series, No. 51, 2003.

165. *Evaluation of certain veterinary drug residues in food* (Sixty-first report of the Joint FAO/WHO Expert Committee on Food Additives). WHO Technical Report Series, No. 922, 2004.

166. *Toxicological evaluation of certain veterinary drug residues in food.* WHO Food Additives Series, No. 52, (in preparation).

Annex 2
Recommendations on compounds on the agenda

Antimicrobial agents

Cefuroxime

Acceptable daily intake:
The temporary ADI established at the fifty-eighth meeting of the Committee (WHO TRS 911, 2002) was withdrawn.

Residues:
The temporary MRL for cows' milk was withdrawn.

Chloramphenicol

Acceptable daily intake:
The Committee concluded that it is not appropriate to establish an ADI for chloramphenicol.

Residues:
The Committee concluded that:

There was no evidence supporting the hypothesis that chloramphenicol is synthesized naturally in detectable amounts in soil. Although this possibility is highly unlikely, data generated with modern analytical methods would be required to confirm this;

There was evidence that low concentrations of chloramphenicol found in food monitoring programmes in the year 2002 could not originate from residues of chloramphenicol persisting in the environment after historical veterinary uses of the drug in food-producing animals. However, owing to the high variability of the half-life of chloramphenicol under different environmental conditions, such a mechanism might occasionally cause low-level contamination in food;

Valid analytical methods are available to monitor low levels of chloramphenicol in foods. However, confirmatory methods require sophisticated and expensive equipment.

Flumequine

Acceptable daily intake:
The Committee re-established an ADI of 0–30 µg/kg bw.

Residue definition:
Flumequine

Recommended maximum residue limits (MRLs)

Species	Fat (µg/kg)	Kidney (µg/kg)	Liver (µg/kg)	Muscle (µg/kg)
Cattle	1000	3000	500	500
Black tiger shrimp (*P. monodon*)	—	—	—	500[a]
Chickens	1000	3000	500	500
Pigs	1000	3000	500	500
Sheep	1000	3000	500	500
Trout	—	—	—	500[b]

[a] The MRL is temporary; the following information is requested by 2006: (1) A detailed description of a regulatory method, including its performance characteristics and validation data; (2) Information on the approved dose for treatment of black tiger shrimp and the results of residue studies conducted at the recommended dose.
[b] Muscle including normal proportions of skin.

Lincomycin

Acceptable daily intake: 0–30 µg/kg bw (established at the fifty-fourth meeting of the Committee (WHO TRS 900, 2001))

Residues: The MRLs that were recommended by the fifty-fourth (WHO TRS 900, 2001) and fifty-eighth (WHO TRS 911, 2002) meetings of the Committee were not reconsidered and were maintained.

MRLs for cattle tissues were considered but not recommended by the Committee at its present meeting.

Pirlimycin

Acceptable daily intake: The Committee established an ADI of 0–8 µg/kg bw

Residue definition: Pirlimycin

Recommended maximum residue limits (MRLs)[a]

Species	Fat (µg/kg)	Kidney (µg/kg)	Liver (µg/kg)	Milk (µg/kg)	Muscle (µg/kg)
Cattle	100	400	1000	100	100

[a] For the maximum residue limits for pirlimycin, the Committee noted that the analytical method submitted by the sponsor had been validated suitably, however, the mass spectrometry interface used was no longer commercially available and therefore the method would not comply with all Codex requirements for a Regulatory Analytical Method. Since the Committee received information that verification of this method using different equipment was in progress, it recommended that CCRVDF should propose the MRL for adoption by the Codex Alimentarius Commission only if this work has been completed and made available to the Working Group Methods of Analysis and Sampling in the CCRVDF.

Insecticides

Cyhalothrin

Acceptable daily intake: 0–5 µg/kg bw

Residues definition: Cyhalothrin

Recommended maximum residue limits (MRLs)

Species	Fat (µg/kg)	Kidney (µg/kg)	Liver (µg/kg)	Milk (µg/kg)	Muscle (µg/kg)
Cattle	400	20	20	30	20
Pigs	400	20	20	—	20
Sheep	400	20	50	—	20

Cypermethrin and α-cypermethrin

Acceptable daily intake: The Committee established a group ADI of 0–20 µg/kg bw for cypermethrin and α-cypermethrin

Residue definition: Total of cypermethrin residues (resulting from the use of cypermethrin or α-cypermethrin as veterinary drugs)

Recommended maximum residue limits (MRLs)

Species	Fat (µg/kg)	Kidney (µg/kg)	Liver (µg/kg)	Milk (µg/kg)	Muscle (µg/kg)
Cattle	1000	50	50	100	50
Sheep	1000	50	50	100	50

Doramectin

Acceptable daily intake: 0–1 µg/kg bw (established at the fifty-eighth meeting of the Committee (WHO TRS 911, 2002))

Residue definition: Doramectin

Recommended maximum residue limit (MRL)

Species	Milk (µg/kg)
Cattle	15[a]

[a] The Committee noted that (1) on the basis of the MRL of 15 mg/kg for doramectin in whole milk from cows, the milk-discard times would be approximately 240 h, according to studies using the pour-on treatment. Milk discard times would be approximately 480 h after treatment with doramectin the dose formulated for injection; (2) in milk containing 4% milk fat, the residues in milk fat would be equivalent to 375 µg/kg (15 µg/kg ÷ 0.04 = 375 µg/kg). This is higher than the MRL of 150 µg/kg in fat tissue; (3) the discard time necessary to accommodate the recommended MRL in milk is unlikely to be consistent with good veterinary practice.

Phoxim

Acceptable daily intake: 0–4 µg/kg bw (established at the fifty-second meeting of the Committee (WHO TRS 893, 2000))

Residues: The MRLs for sheep, pigs and goats that were recommended by the Committee at its fifty-eighth meeting (WHO TRS 911, 2002) were not reconsidered and were maintained.

The temporary MRLs for cattle that were recommended by theCommittee at its fifty-second (WHO TRS 893, 2000) and fifty-eighth (WHO TRS 911, 2002) meetings were withdrawn.

Production aids

Melengestrol acetate

Acceptable daily intake: 0–0.03 µg/kg bw (established at the fifty-fourth meeting of the Committee (WHO TRS 900, 2001)

Residues definition: Melengestrol acetate

Recommended maximum residue limits (MRLs)

Species	Fat (µg/kg)	Liver (µg/kg)
Cattle	8	5

Ractopamine

Acceptable daily intake: 0–1 µg/kg bw

Residues definition: Ractopamine

Recommended maximum residue limits (MRLs)

Species	Fat (µg/kg)	Kidney (µg/kg)	Liver (µg/kg)	Muscle (µg/kg)
Cattle	10	90	40	10
Pigs	10	90	40	10